Looking Back (and Forth)

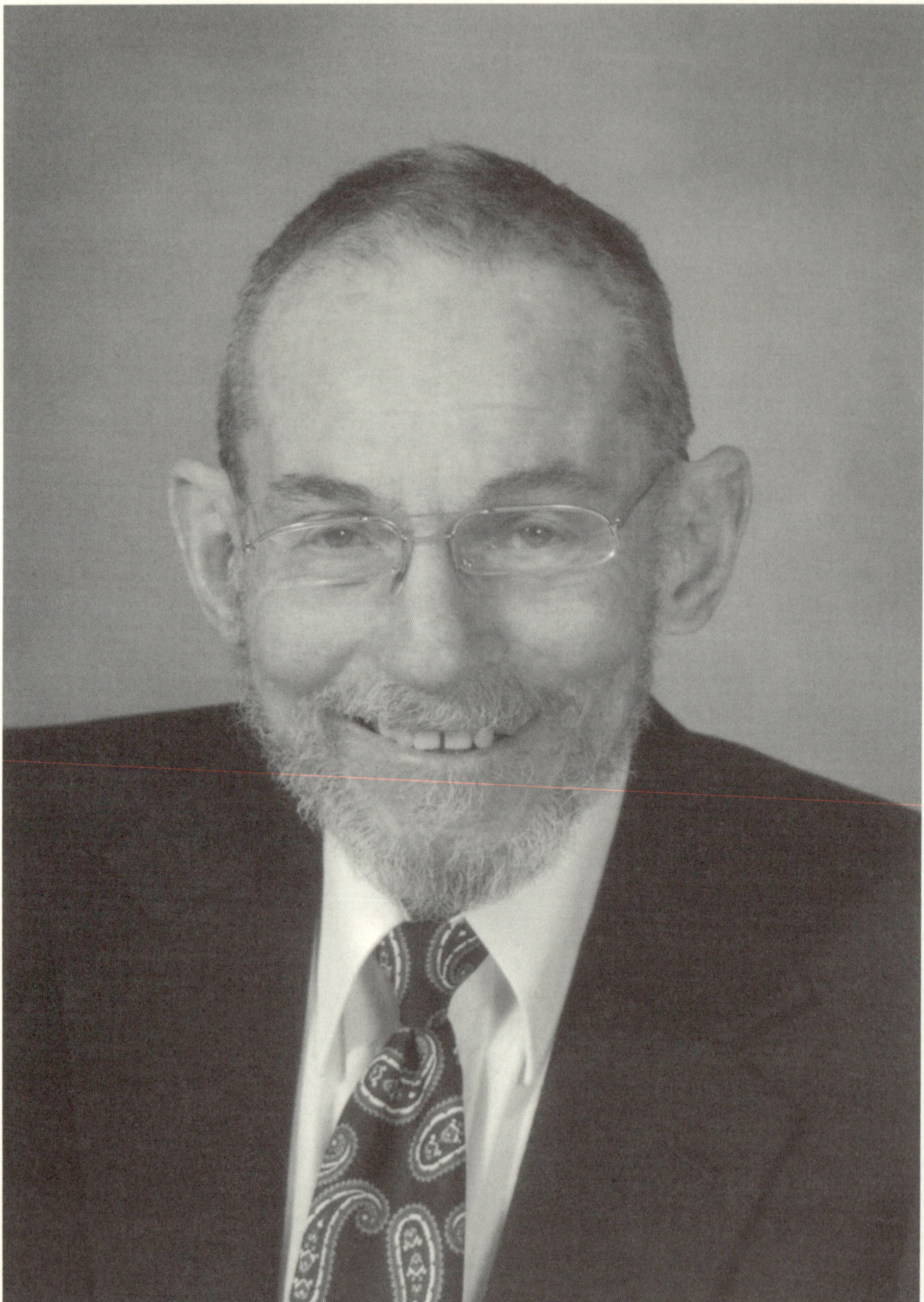

Looking Back (and Forth)

Reflections of an Old-Fashioned Doctor

Herbert L. Fred, M.D.

Professor of Medicine
University of Texas Health Science Center at Houston
and
Clinical Director, Department of Medicine
Lyndon B. Johnson General Hospital
Houston, Texas

Mercer
University
Press

ISBN 0-86554-772-6
MUP/H583

6316 Peake Road
Macon, Georgia 31210-3960

First Edition.

∞The paper used in this publication meets the minimum requirements of American National Standard for Information Sciences—Permanence of Paper for Printed Library Materials, ANSI Z39.48-1992.

Library of Congress Cataloging-in-Publication Data

Fred, Herbert L.
Looking back (and forth) : reflections of an old-fashioned doctor / Herbert L. Fred.— 1st ed.
p. cm.
ISBN 0-86554-772-6 (hbk. : alk. paper)
1. Medicine—Miscellanea. I. Title.
R708.F837 2003
610—dc21

2003003678

Contents

In loving memory of bedside medicine

Foreword

"[T]he practice of medicine is an art, not a trade."
–William Osler

In today's highly technological environment, physicians can easily get so caught up in the science of medicine that they tend to neglect the art of medicine. However, the physician's role is not solely that of a scientist but also that of a caregiver and humanitarian. Today's physicians must find a balance between the traditions of the past (which emphasized empathy, compassion, and direct patient care) and the policies of the present (which place a premium on sophisticated machines and gadgets).

In this volume of collected articles, Dr. Herbert L. Fred questions many of today's medical practices. He urges physicians to hold fast to the patient-oriented traditions that have sustained our profession throughout its history. He reminds us that "newer" does not always mean "better." He insists that physicians must continue to value conventional diagnostic tools such as a thorough patient history and physical examination. He stresses the importance of sound management, based on a proper initial diagnosis, as well as careful follow-up evaluation.

Dr. Fred is not a technophobe, nor is his book a preachy diatribe. His humorous style and liberal use of anecdotes make the book lively and entertaining. Originally published in *Hospital Practice, Southern Medical Journal,* and *Houston Medicine,* these essays are just the right length to be read in spare moments. Because each one is complete in itself, they do not need to be read in any particular order.

The author of two previous books, Dr. Fred has published hundreds of medical articles and is on the editorial boards of several medical journals. As a professor in the Department of Internal Medicine at The University of Texas Health Science Center (Houston), he has devoted his life to educating young physicians. Over the years, he has been in great demand as a writer and speaker.

He has also been involved in sports medicine and has broken many records as a long-distance runner. This may be one reason why he has such a long perspective as a medical philosopher.

I commend Dr. Fred for his wit, sagacity, clinical acumen, and ability with words. Having balanced the art and science of medicine in an exemplary manner, he is a role model for us all.

Denton A. Cooley, M.D.
Surgeon-in-Chief
Texas Heart Institute
Houston

Foreword

I am a young physician, now thirty-two years old, and in private practice in the Piney Woods of East Texas. In my life, I have been fortunate enough to know a few great men. Only one of them will be legendary.

Part of my fourth year in medical school was spent under the tutelage of this legend, Dr. Herb Fred, learning the qualities that separate one doctor from another. As I moved on to other teachers, other places, his voice remained fixed in my conscience, objecting to my sloth, indifference, and fear, but also encouraging and exhorting. Looking back, I realize his style is the kind that makes a difference in outstanding patient care.

He views medicine as an art that must be practiced and improved upon daily: learned and relearned. And he hammers into his residents the concept that perfect practice is not a once-in-a-while thing but something that must be done all the time. I now see my time with Dr. Fred as a surge in my understanding of the power of curiosity, the importance of individuality, and the reasons why we must be committed to an unwavering honesty in medicine. Under him, I learned to abandon my obsequious and dewy-eyed view of authority and embrace skepticism as a trait of a good doctor. One can easily find these sentiments reflected in his writing.

In the pages of this book, as well as his others, Dr. Fred exhorts us to move off "high-center" and act, or choose decisively to wait; he leads us to attend the sick and relieve their suffering, not to triage them mindlessly into the appropriate algorithm of treatment and discharge planning; to continue to think—even after a diagnosis is made—and not be lulled to sleep, then caught off guard by the flux of disease, the vacillations of recovery and relapse. We are to develop a sense of urgency and purpose in our daily routine.

These habits aren't universally popular, nor do they come easily. They are hard and lonely rules to live by, and as technology lumbers forward, people are increasingly unaware of the role these traits must play if patients are to receive quality care. No physician is ever thanked for watchful waiting or for performing an appropriately complete examination rather than one to simply satisfy proper billing. Rather, one is rewarded with the quiet satisfaction of having done the task laid in front with "all your heart, soul, mind, and strength."

Dr. Fred illuminates the issues a good physician wrestles with daily, the weaknesses one struggles to overcome, when deciding to do the right thing. His example and precepts continue to help me chisel myself into the kind of physician I want to be.

Patrick T. Russell, M.D.

Acknowledgments

A book is never the work of one individual. To paraphrase Hillary Rodham Clinton, it takes a village to produce a book. In that light, I wish to thank the following villagers: Mark Scheid, Ph.D., of Rice University, who serves as my writing mentor; Kenneth E. Sack, M.D., Professor of Clinical Medicine, University of California, San Francisco, for his priceless critiques of my manuscripts; John B. Thomison, M.D., former Editor, *Southern Medical Journal,* and Lee Powers, former Executive Editor, *Hospital Practice,* for publishing many of the essays assembled here; Sue Robinson and Darlene Makransky for their secretarial assistance; and Susan Carini, Director of Publications, Emory University, for her advice, encouragement, and general savvy.

And finally, I thank God for my wife, Judy. Of my many blessings, she tops the list.

Original Publication Sources

The essays in this book, except for "Looking Back" (pp 95-99), were published previously in various medical journals and are reprinted here with full permission from those journals. The original publication sources are listed below.

Old-Fashioned Doctors. Hosp Pract 33:15, December 1998.

I Remember When. South Med J 85:1242-43, December 1992.

The Tyranny of Technology. Hosp Pract 32:17-21, March 15, 1997.

Tenets for Physicians in the New Millenium. Hosp Pract 35:13-16, February 15, 2000.

Just What the Doctor Ordered. Hosp Pract 34:11-12, December 15, 1999.

Remember the Rattlesnake. Hosp Pract 34:7-8, July 15, 1999.

Washing Our Hands of the Matter. Hosp Pract 34:11, March 15, 1999.

Digital Rectal Examination During Early Acute MI. Hosp Pract 32:15-16, September 15, 1997.

The Interesting Patient. Hosp Pract 28:10, April 15, 1993.

Algorithms: Let's Give Them Back. Hosp Pract 35:15-16, September 15, 2000.

The Numbers Game. Hosp Pract 35:11-16, July 15, 2000.

Doing Nothing. South Med J 85:343, April 1992.

Previous Medical Records: Lest We Forget. Hosp Pract 29:79-87, July 15, 1994.

The Blind Leading the Blind. Hosp Pract 35:12-15, May 15, 2000.

Requiem for the Ophthalmoscope. Hosp Pract 29:37-38, February 15, 1994.

Night Sweats. Hosp Pract 28:88, August 15, 1993.

To Be *B* or Not to Be *B*—Is That the Question? Tex Heart Inst J 29:1-2, 2002.

The Shakespearean Principle. Hosp Pract 33:83-84, September 15, 1998.

Curable Conspicuous Ascites: The Forgotten Four. Hosp Pract 34:98-100, October 15, 1999.

When the Bell Doesn't Ring. Hosp Pract 32:54, November 15, 1997.

Five Cases in Search of a Diagnostician. Hosp Pract 28:72-76, April 30, 1993.

Courvoisier Revisited. Houston Medicine 8:65-66, September 1992.

Contarini's Condition. South Med J 85:33-34, January 1992.

The Clinicopathological Conference. Hosp Pract 33:11-16, October 15, 1998.

DLTBGYD. Hosp Pract 34:15-16, October 15, 1999.

Dizzy Medical Writing and Editing: No Relief in Sight. South Med J 85:743-745, July 1992.

Dizzy Medical Writing and Editing: A Decade of Non-Progress. South Med J 86:705-709, June 1993.

Dizzy Medical Editing: Causes, Consequences, and Cures. South Med J 84:760-762, June 1991.

On Being Politically Correct. South Med J 85:865, September 1992.

Clinical Observations During a 1,000-Mile Footrace. Houston Medicine 5:38-42, June 1989.

On An Average Day. Houston Medicine 8:1, March 1992.

Parliament of Whores. South Med J 84:1, January 1992.

Cause or Coincidence? South Med J 85:923, September 1992.

There But for the Grace of God. . . Houston Medicine 8:38-39, June 1992.

C. T. Scanner Dies. Hosp Pract 36:23, January 15, 2001.

CARING FOR THE PATIENT

And I believe that if more doctors today practiced medicine the old-fashioned way, our profession might regain some of the nobility and respect it once enjoyed.

–H. L. F. in "Old-Fashioned Doctors"

Treat your patient, not yourself.

–H. L. F. in "Just What the Doctor Ordered"

A serious malady pervades and undermines our profession. I call it the numbers game—treating a number (or some test result) rather than the patient who has that number.

–H. L. F. in "The Numbers Game"

Old-Fashioned Doctors

In the forty years that I have been a full-time medical educator, much has changed regarding what we teach and how we teach our students and house officers. As a consequence, I now confine myself to teaching basic medical principles—principles that should never change. But even so, today's trainees tell me that what I say and do is old-fashioned. I wonder:

—Is it because old-fashioned doctors spend whatever time it takes to obtain a good medical history and physical examination?

—Is it because old-fashioned doctors routinely seek *all* of the patient's previous medical records, not just the discharge summaries?

—Is it because old-fashioned doctors do not order sophisticated, expensive studies when simpler and cheaper procedures can supply the needed information?

—Is it because old-fashioned doctors order tests to substantiate, not generate, their clinical impressions?

—Is it because old-fashioned doctors use their brain and their heart, not an army of consultants, to manage their patients?

—Is it because old-fashioned doctors view consultants as opinion givers, not decision makers?

—Is it because old-fashioned doctors treat patients, not numbers?

—Is it because old-fashioned doctors do not blindly administer a ton of drugs in an attempt to alleviate every possible ill?
—Is it because old-fashioned doctors recognize that doing nothing is, at times, doing a lot?
—Is it because old-fashioned doctors understand that patients often get well *despite* what we do, not as a result of what we do?
—Is it because old-fashioned doctors realize that good rapport with their patients is the best protection against lawsuits?
—Is it because old-fashioned doctors are aware of their own fallibility and are never afraid to say, "I don't know"?

If so, then I am proud to be old-fashioned. And I believe that if more doctors today practiced medicine the old-fashioned way, our profession might regain some of the nobility and respect it once enjoyed.

I Remember When

Medicine has undergone many changes—so many, in fact, that I find myself looking back these days much more than I look ahead. Perhaps it's just a sign of aging. I now enjoy senior citizen discounts on airline tickets, and next year I'll be eligible for Medicare. Whatever the reason, reflecting on Medicine as I once knew it brings me a sense of pleasure and satisfaction. And from such reflection, I have a better perspective on Medicine as we practice it today.

I remember when:

—House officers had no formal contracts; unless they demonstrated unflagging commitment, they were fired.

—Compensation for interns ranged from room and board only to (as in my case) $50 a month.

—Interns worked every day and at least every other night, all year long.

—Medical students, interns, or both did all of the initial and follow-up blood counts, urinalyses, stool guaiac tests, sputum stains, and electrocardiograms.

—Interns on call drew morning blood samples from all of the ward patients—usually about thirty, sometimes more.

—Intensive Care and Coronary Care Units were nonexistent, and life-support equipment was crude.

—Monitoring seriously ill patients required use of one's mind and five senses, coupled with frequent trips to the bedside and long bedside vigils.

—Pacemakers were bigger than car batteries, were housed next to the patient's bed, and with each electrical impulse, the patient's entire body jumped.
—Intravenous fluids were made in the hospital and administered through reusable rubber tubing.
—Southey tubes were inserted subcutaneously to relieve intractable peripheral edema.
—Syringes were made of glass, and needles were not disposable.
—Serum potassium levels and blood gas determinations were available only from research laboratories, and only once or twice a week.
—Measuring the venous pressure in the antecubital space and determining the circulation time were standard procedures for all cardiac patients.
—Rheumatic heart disease was almost as common as coronary artery disease.
—Syphilitic aneurysm of the thoracic aorta was a leading cause of superior vena cava syndrome.
—Poliomyelitis was rampant, and patients in "iron lungs" occupied much of the physician's time.
—Weekly grand rounds consisted of two or three case presentations in which the patients were there in person for everyone to see and for a privileged few to question and examine.
—Autopsies were an indispensable teaching tool, required for hospital accreditation.
—Radiologists wore red goggles.
—Only the attending physician wrote orders for the patient.
—Physicians sought consultations to gain new information or a new perspective, not to save time and thought, protect against litigation, or repay colleagues for previous favors.
—Referring physicians and consultants met at the bedside to examine patients together.

—Consultants rendered opinions, not mandates.
—The primary physician always remained in charge of the patient's care.
—House calls were part of the practitioner's daily routine.
—Health insurance was affordable and easy to get.
—Medical malpractice suits were virtually unheard of, and lawyers were physicians' friends.
—Taking a good medical history and doing a careful physical examination were coveted skills.
—An ECHO was something you might hear after shouting in a canyon, MRI referred to moderate renal insufficiency, and a CAT scan meant stealing a glimpse of your feline pet.

I remember when Medicine was a highly respected calling, the noblest of professions.

The Tyranny of Technology

During the past twenty years or so, advances in medical technology have greatly enhanced our ability to diagnose and treat disease. For example, now that we have computed tomography (CT), we no longer rely on intravenous urography or retroperitoneal air insufflation to assess adrenal size; we no longer fill the stomach and intestines with barium to detect pancreatic masses; and we no longer make six burr holes in the skull to exclude subdural hematoma. Similarly, the advent of magnetic resonance imaging (MRI), ultrasonography, and transesophageal echocardiography has enabled us to establish diagnoses with speed, accuracy, and safety never before dreamed of.

But too much of something good often leads to something bad. And from my view as a full-time medical educator for almost four and a half decades, I do, indeed, see something bad. I call it "technologic tenesmus," the uncontrollable urge to rely on sophisticated medical gadgetry for diagnoses.

Technologic tenesmus pervades our profession and has reached epidemic proportions. It is insidious in onset, highly contagious, and rapidly addictive. All of us are endangered, particularly the ill-trained or ill-informed, and those looking for shortcuts, fearing litigation, or lacking in self-confidence. Unaware of their affliction, the victims become tools of the laboratory—shackled to the routine of using advanced technology to *formulate* rather than to *verify* their clinical impressions.

Tyranny in Action

Overreliance on sophisticated gadgetry can lead to bad outcomes in at least *three* different ways, as the following cases illustrate.

First, the gadget is broken or unavailable when needed.

CASE 1. A forty-year-old alcoholic woman presented with high fever and altered sensorium of several hours' duration. On examination, she was delirious, tremulous, diaphoretic, and icteric with no localizing neurologic signs and with normal optic discs.

Among the many diagnostic possibilities, bacterial meningitis, intracranial hemorrhage or hematoma, and delirium tremens were major concerns. Accordingly, I recommended immediate lumbar puncture. The attending physician, however, disagreed. His reason? "Conventional wisdom."

"Before we do a lumbar puncture," he said, "we must get a CT scan. Otherwise, she could herniate."

"Given this patient's history and physical findings," I replied, "the benefits of a lumbar puncture infinitely outweigh any of the theoretical risks."

Approximately five hours after our conversation, the attending physician learned that the CT scanner was not in service. He then decided to treat the patient empirically with antibiotics. Four more hours elapsed before the patient finally received the CT scan followed by a lumbar puncture. (Fortunately, the results of both studies were normal.)

In this case, there was a five-hour delay in starting empirical antibiotic therapy and a nine-hour delay in withdrawing spinal fluid for analysis—all because the CT scanner was not operative.

Second, the gadget is working but gives normal or inconclusive findings.

CASE 2. A thirty-two-year-old woman had acute hemiplegia. In presenting the case to me, the resident said, "The CT scan of this patient's head is negative, and I don't know what to do next."

Had the resident taken a social history, she would have discovered serious marital turmoil. Had she been more observant, she would have noticed the patient's histrionic behavior. And had she done a more careful neurologic examination, she would have found the hemiplegia to vary when the patient's attention was directed elsewhere. Even the patient's husband suggested the right diagnosis: "I think it's all in her head," he opined.

Computed tomography is a wonderful device, but it cannot detect hysteria.

Third, the gadget gives conclusive, abnormal findings that prompt inappropriate intervention.

CASE 3. A forty-six-year-old man with sprue underwent exploratory celiotomy for suspected perforated bowel. A CT scan of his abdomen had shown free air beneath his diaphragm and in the colonic wall. In reviewing the case, I determined that at the time of celiotomy, the patient had minimal abdominal discomfort and his physical examination was unremarkable. The operation disclosed air in the retroperitoneum, mesentery, and colonic wall but showed no visceral perforation. In retrospect, findings on the preoperative plain abdominal film were diagnostic of pneumatosis cystoides intestinalis, a well-established cause of spontaneous pneumoperitoneum without signs of peritonitis. The preoperative chest film also showed free air beneath the diaphragm.

This case, as in many others I've seen, is an excellent example of treating a laboratory value, not the patient. It also illustrates another common manifestation of technologic tenesmus—ordering a sophisticated study when cheaper, conventional tests have already supplied sufficient information.

What Can Be Done?

Is there a cure for this malady of practice, this tyranny of technology? Many believe that the cost-containment policies of managed care companies will bring about the needed changes. Maybe so, but I don't see that as the solution. The motive of managed care companies has little to do with altruism or clinical excellence. These companies reduce the indiscriminate use of expensive tests and procedures, but they also deny appropriate requests for the same studies. Furthermore, their policies don't address the basic cause of technologic tenesmus—inadequate physician education.

Lasting reversal or amelioration of technologic tenesmus would require, at a minimum, the revamping of our medical school teaching faculties. Currently, these faculties consist largely of two groups: fellows and young instructors who are fact-filled but experience-thin, and older professors who are proficient in only a narrow segment of their specialty. Both groups spend most of their time lecturing, writing papers, working in the clinics or laboratory, or traveling to meetings. These activities, whether school-decreed or self-imposed, limit contact between the faculty and trainees. Teaching takes place more often in the lecture hall, conference room, or hallway outside the patient's room than at the patient's bedside. Consequently, students and house officers spend more and more time attending lectures or conferences and less and less time attending patients. Having little direct access to the teaching staff, the trainees turn to house officers only one or two years their senior for much of their instruction. Complicating matters further, most of today's teachers received their training in the technologic era. No wonder they favor high-tech medicine. They've never learned the high-touch approach.

We need more teachers who learned to make diagnoses by understanding the pathophysiology, clinical features, and natural history of diseases. Most—but not all—of these physicians trained at a time when MRI referred to moderate renal insufficiency, and an "echo" was only something you might hear after shouting in a canyon. They know what tests, if any, to order, when to order them, and how to interpret them. And they use advanced technology to *verify* rather than to *formulate* their clinical impressions.

These are the teachers who truly comprehend the value of a good medical history, the rewards of a pertinent physical examination, and the power of knowing how to think. These are the teachers who still routinely use the stethoscope, not an echocardiogram, to detect valvular heart disease; who use the ophthalmoscope, not magnetic resonance imaging, to detect intracranial hypertension; who use their eyes, not a blood gas apparatus, to detect cyanosis; who use their hands, not computed tomography, to detect splenomegaly; and who use their brain and their heart, not a horde of consultants, to manage their patients.

And these are the teachers who don't order expensive, state-of-the-art studies when cheaper, conventional tests supply the same information; who don't administer a slew of medications in an effort to alleviate every possible ill; who appreciate that doing nothing is, at times, doing a lot; and who realize that many patients get well despite what we do, not because of what we do.

Unfortunately, these necessary role models are a vanishing species. Most of them have died or retired, and those who still have regular contact with medical students and house officers are too few to stem the tide of technologic tenesmus.

Can we possibly replenish these role models? I don't think so. But even if we could, it wouldn't be enough. We need to take advantage of the role models currently practicing good medicine outside of academia. What these practitioners see and do each day bears scant resemblance to what students and house officers see and do in the hospital and lecture hall. Therefore, a good part of the trainee's clinical experience should take place in the real-world setting, supervised by experienced, compassionate, commonsense doctors.

Finally, we need to take our monitoring system away from lawyers and insurance companies and put it where it belongs—with us. If we can truly develop and implement an equitable way of keeping ourselves in line, a cure for technologic tenesmus may then become possible.

Tenets for Physicians in the New Millennium

Dear Dad,

It has been months since I left for college, and I've been remiss in writing. Nevertheless, I'm getting along fine now. The skull fracture I got when I jumped out of the window when my dormitory caught on fire is pretty well healed. Fortunately, an attendant at the gas station near the dorm saw me jump. And since I had nowhere to live after the fire, he kindly invited me to share his basement room. He's a fine boy and we have fallen deeply in love and plan to get married. We haven't set the date yet, but it will be before my pregnancy begins to show. I know you'll welcome him even though his religion is different from ours.

Now that I've brought you up to date, I want to tell you that there was no dormitory fire. I didn't have a concussion or skull fracture, I'm not pregnant, and there isn't any man in my life. But I am getting a D in History and an F in Algebra, and I wanted you to see those marks in their proper perspective.

Your loving daughter...

Hooray for that college student. Her letter points out something we all know but too frequently forget: There's more to an education than academics.

As a full-time medical educator for the past four decades, I am encountering an increasing number of house officers who score well on written tests but are woefully inept at the bedside. To be a competent physician, one needs much more than book knowledge. In fact, some of the most important information in the medical literature has little to do with science *per se.* Consider, for example, the following:

Learning Medicine

Learning the best way to learn medicine is something many physicians never learn. George T. Harrell, when dean at the University of Florida College of Medicine, suggested that "The physician's continuing education...is largely a process within himself, one he pursues on his own...[M]ost of his true learning—the part that sticks with him—is what he does for himself, by himself."

Joseph Sapira, physical diagnostician extraordinaire, addressed learning in relation to his "ectopic brain"—a collection of notes he used for solving clinical problems. After he had amassed a thick set of these notes, his students began asking permission to photocopy them. "[T]he wickedest thing I have done is to make available a prepackaged ectopic brain involving no work on the part of the student. The crux of the personal ectopic brain is that it requires one to learn how to teach one's self. To me this is the most important, perhaps the only mandatory lesson of a medical education. By providing a completed version of the thing, I have deprived the student of the opportunity to make his own and so have enucleated his education."

Leonard K. Nash, an award-winning chemist, offered this: "Teachers don't teach; at most they stir students to learn. Teachers promote learning less by the answers they give than by the questions they raise.... The most active role in education belongs not to the teacher but to the student."

Amen!

Seeking Excellence

To rise above the norm of mediocrity, one must strive diligently for excellence. In that light, Raymond Pruitt, one-time chairman of the department of medicine, Baylor University College of Medicine, said, "Excellence, wherever sought, is not easily found. Its possession requires a mind quick to discernment of flaws, a nature intolerant of needless error, a will unbending in pursuit of high accomplishment."

William Bean, a giant of internal medicine during his lifetime, summarized it this way: "There is no magic vitamin, no capsule of intellectual chemotherapy, which will serve in the place of the one medicine which gives excellence—hard work."

Being Honest

A highly respected surgeon, Oscar Creech, Jr., wrote, "None of us likes to appear ignorant nor do we enjoy being in error. The senior medical student feels that he must answer the questions of freshmen and sophomores or he isn't worthy of his high position. The senior resident, idol of medical students, interns, and assistant residents, hesitates to say 'I don't know' or 'It was a mistake to operate on that patient' or 'I completely missed the diagnosis,' for he might quickly lose his following.... And so, a confused reply is given, an error in diagnosis rationalized, an operative mishap covered up. [And] the young physician...has suddenly become aware that a mediocre performance can be made to appear first-rate if presented properly."

Two synergistic factors are paramount in causing dishonesty in medicine. One is a background of intense competition. We compete to get into medical school; we compete to stay there; and we compete for the internship and residency of our choice. Thereafter, we compete for patients, research grants, and the like.

The other factor is human frailty, especially ignorance, greed, fear of being wrong, and the need for aggrandizement. Patients frequently foster these frailties by conferring godlike qualities on us. In return, we prevaricate to protect this image for them as well as for our colleagues and ourselves. Though dishonesty is sometimes a matter of interpretation, condoning or forgiving it is unacceptable—and in the field of medicine, can be tragic.

Avoiding Arrogance

Franz Ingelfinger, former editor of *The New England Journal of Medicine*, maintained that "many physicians are indeed arrogant in their behavior toward patients...." He argued, however, that in some cases, a physician could be beneficially arrogant if paternalism and dominance were used appropriately. But he also said, "Doctors for various reasons find it difficult to put themselves in the patient's place; they do not sufficiently appreciate, or perhaps do not have the time to appreciate, how the patient feels and how he reacts to the medical information and procedures to which he is exposed."

I agree that arrogance among physicians is common and believe that it has several causes. As a group, we are intelligent, have an inordinate amount of schooling and training, routinely render important decisions regarding the lives of our fellow human beings, and characteristically answer only to ourselves. Consequently, we can easily become haughty and egocentric, with a false sense of omnipotence. But our arrogance often is a front for ignorance and insecurity and can crumble as knowledge builds. We can also fight any godlike tendencies with an "anti-deiotic"—a mixture of humility and honesty.

Promoting Skepticism

According to Joseph Alpert and Robert Coles, "Skepticism is a philosophical state of mind essential to the scientific method and to the modern practice of medicine. Ironically and not rarely, skepticism in medical education is often in jeopardy—a victim of authoritative opinions, handed down in the name of 'science.' Young physicians in training can be especially vulnerable to such a development and can become all too unskeptical as they sit and gobble up plate after plate of factuality. Meanwhile, a skeptical approach to knowledge is rarely taught, either in medical school or during postgraduate medical education. At the present time, medical school and postgraduate medical programs often stifle skeptical attitudes among student and graduate physicians."

Maxwell Wintrobe, my mentor and a world-renowned hematologist, expressed similar sentiments. "To my mind," he said, "science owes its success to doubting all things.... Too many physicians are willing to ride with the tide, to follow the flood of undigested literature and to be carried away by the claims of the uncritical."

In academia, we usually embrace whatever the professor says or whatever the textbook or medical journal declares. We don't always realize or remember that another professor, another journal, or another text may put an entirely different spin on the same subject. History, both medical and general, is filled with stories of individuals who tried to introduce new ideas but couldn't penetrate the party line. This barrier continues to produce blind acquiescence and stifled innovation.

Serving Our Patients

In 1927, Francis Peabody, professor of medicine at Harvard Medical School, penned *the* classic article on this subject. His words ring true today as they did then and as they will for years to come. Note these excerpts:

"Medicine is not a trade to be learned but a profession to be entered."

"[I]t is one thing to write an examination paper on treating gastric ulcer and quite another thing to treat John Smith, who happens to have a gastric ulcer."

"[P]hysicians, by wrong diagnoses and ill-considered statements, are responsible for many wrecked lives, and you will discover that it is much easier to make a wrong diagnosis than it is to 'unmake' it."

"The good physician knows his patients through and through, and his knowledge is bought dearly. Time, sympathy, and understanding must be lavishly dispensed, but the reward is to be found in that personal bond which forms the greatest satisfaction of the practice of medicine. One of the essential qualities of the clinician is interest in humanity, for the secret of the care of the patient is in caring *for* the patient."

Coda

What lies ahead for medicine in the new millennium is any-body's guess. In the foreseeable future, however, nothing is likely to supplant the tenets for physicians cited here—tenets that have already served humankind well for several millennia.

Selected Reading

Alpert JS, Coles R. Loss of skepticism in medical education. Arch Intern Med 149:2637, 1989.

Bean WB. Convocation Comments. J Iowa State Med Soc 40:22, 1950.

Creech O Jr. The voice of the cricket. Bull Tulane Univ Med Faculty 17:53, 1957.

Harrell GT. Traditional vs. novel approaches to medical education. J Med Educ 33 (Oct, Pt II): 217, 1958.

Ingelfinger FJ. Arrogance. N Engl J Med 303:1507, 1980.

Nash LK. Concerning teachees. *In* Hippocrates Revisited: A Search for Meaning, Bulger RJ (Ed). Medcom Press, New York, 1973, pp 213–215.

Peabody FW. The care of the patient. JAMA 88:877, 1927.

Pruitt RD. On being almost right. Cardiovasc Res Center Bull 2:34, 1963.

Sapira JD. A personal history of the ectopic brain. South Med J 83:1203, 1990.

Wintrobe MM. The virtue of doubt and the spirit of inquiry. Trans Assoc Amer Phys 78:1, 1965.

Just What the Doctor Ordered

What would you say is the most important component of the inpatient medical record? I recently put that question to a group of medical students, house officers, and senior clinicians in the department of internal medicine at a university teaching hospital. To promote unencumbered responses, I forewarned each participant that my question has no right or wrong answer.

Almost immediately, all thirteen medical students, twelve of the seventeen house officers, and eight of the ten senior clinicians picked the history and physical examination. Just as quickly, two house officers selected the nurses' notes, and one clinician chose the progress notes. The remaining clinician and three house officers hesitated a bit, thought aloud, then settled on the doctors' orders.

Clearly, *all* components of the inpatient medical record are important. I devised my question, however, to test my belief that most physicians take the doctors' order sheet for granted.

Think about it this way: The care that any hospitalized patient receives—be it good or otherwise—ultimately depends on what the doctor orders, how those orders are interpreted, and when and how they are implemented. Yet, formal instruction in order-writing has never been part of the medical school curriculum and probably never will be. Furthermore, the medical literature and standard medical textbooks devote little attention to the subject. And few attending physicians regularly critique house officers' orders. Consequently, medical students and house officers "learn" order-writing from each other—the "see-one, do-one, teach-one" method. No wonder only four of forty (10 percent) respondents ranked doctors' orders as the most important component of the inpatient medical record.

Rankings aside, I propose the following rules for order writing:

1. Think before you write. Because what you are about to write is so important, put your thoughts in order before you order.

2. Write legibly. In a study of handwritten orders from 47 staff physicians in a 500-bed teaching hospital, the handwriting was completely illegible in eight (17 percent) orders and barely legible in another eight. Thus, fully one third of these physicians were risking a ticket to the courtroom. If you can't write legibly, print.

3. Do not abbreviate. Abbreviating an order breeds misinterpretation, and the consequences are sometimes devastating. I know of two cases in which a misinterpreted abbreviation led directly to the patient's death. Remember, the only person who invariably knows what an abbreviation stands for is the one who uses it.

4. Be specific. A common written order at my hospital reads "bld cx × 2". This order (for two blood cultures) is bad not only because it is abbreviated (leaving room for confusion) but also because it leaves the time interval up to the nurse. Given such an order, some of our nurses draw just one large sample of blood and place it in two sets of culture tubes. Other nurses arbitrarily draw two samples thirty minutes apart. Writing out "blood cultures" and specifying the exact time each culture specimen should be obtained will eliminate any confusion and guesswork.

5. Be cost- and safety-conscious. Afraid of missing the diagnosis, many physicians order a multitude of tests and an army of consultants. This practice is haphazard, time-consuming, unduly expensive, and occasionally dangerous.

6. Treat your patient, not yourself. An intern wrote an order for "strict I's & O's" (intake and output) on the record of a twenty-five-year-old healthy-appearing woman with cough and an apical infiltrate on her chest x-ray. When I asked him his reason for the order, he replied, "I like to have I's and O's on all of my new patients." What *he* wanted was not what his patient needed.

7. Don't put the cart before the horse. A sixty-two-year-old woman had acute pleurisy and a large, rounded infiltrate in her left lower lobe. Thinking that the patient had lung cancer, the resident ordered a slew of studies to stage it. The "cancer," however, disappeared with antibiotic therapy.

8. Avoid routines. Individualizing your patient's care can save a lot of wasted time, effort, and money. For example, not all hospitalized patients need their temperature, pulse, respiration, and blood pressure checked every six to eight hours. But such orders are routine virtually everywhere. Additionally, not all patients with fever and cough need their sputum stained and cultured for acid-fast and fungal organisms. But orders to that effect are disappointingly common, especially in teaching hospitals.

9. Respect the nursing staff. Many nurses are reluctant to seek clarification of an order because the physician's response all too frequently is abusive (e.g., "Can't you read?" or "Don't bother me, I'm busy" or something even more insulting). As a result, the order may be carried out incorrectly—or not at all. So, if the nurse questions you, be appreciative, and respond accordingly.

10. Be courteous. "Please" and "thank you" are words that rarely find their way onto the doctor's order sheet. But when they do, they do wonders for the nurse-doctor relationship—which in turn benefits the patient.

Regardless of the format used for order-writing, adhering to these rules will go a long way towards maximizing patient care while minimizing patient risks and expense. It will also protect physicians against lawsuits. In fact, it should be just what the doctor ordered.

Selected Reading

Anonymous. A study of physicians' handwriting as a time-waster. JAMA 242:2429, 1979.

Lesar TS et al. Medication prescribing errors in a teaching hospital. JAMA 263:2329, 1990.

Thai, HM. Writing orders for hospitalized patients. *In* Clinical Medicine, 2nd edn, Greene HL et al (Eds). Mosby, St. Louis, 1996, pp 52–55.

Remember the Rattlesnake

Assume that you are called to the emergency department to care for a new patient. When you enter the patient's room, you see in the bed a six-foot diamondback rattlesnake, coiled and ready to strike. Since you are now in charge of this "patient," what would you do?

I suspect, and certainly hope, that you would step back, assess your options, and proceed with caution—purposefully contemplating every move you might make. You'd be a fool if you didn't.

The point is this: Good care for some patients calls for the same degree of circumspection required when handling a rattlesnake. Failure to heed this principle does a disservice to the patient and invites trouble for the physician. The trick, therefore, is to recognize the diverse situations in which such circumspection is paramount. Consider the following examples:

CASE 1. A former movie actress complained of fever of four years' duration. She had gone to many physicians in different cities, submitting on each occasion to virtually the same diagnostic procedures and receiving the same types of treatment—all to no avail. During the interview, she talked incessantly, appeared tense, and smoked cigarettes constantly. Her physical findings and results of routine laboratory studies were normal.

Because the history suggested factitious disease, the patient was admitted to the hospital for close observation. It did not take long to catch her putting the lighted end of a cigarette to her thermometer.

Comment. Every time this woman contacted a physician, her "fever" triggered the same response—an array of referrals, myriad tests, and a multitude of therapeutic trials. Four years passed before someone put the case in perspective and stopped the medical merry-go-round.

CASE 2. A thirty-five-year-old woman underwent a right nephrectomy for hypernephroma. Nine years later, she was treated for carcinoma of the cervix. She remained well until age forty-seven when she sustained a 30-lb weight loss. Her gynecologist admitted her to the hospital for evaluation. His examination disclosed signs of weight loss, a palpable liver edge, and mild anemia. He told her that she had advanced cancer and referred her for chemotherapy.

A more detailed medical history uncovered recent heat intolerance and palpitations. On physical examination, the patient had tachycardia, warm skin, a stare, and a diffusely enlarged thyroid. The diagnosis of thyrotoxicosis was made and she received radioactive iodine therapy. When last seen, she was asymptomatic and free of evident disease.

Comment. This case exemplifies the pitfalls of a prejudiced viewpoint—that is, allowing the knowledge of a previously established diagnosis to bias the physician's evaluation of the patient's current illness. Even worse, the physician presumed that the patient had a new, irreversible disease, when in reality she had a curable disease.

CASE 3. An elderly woman complained of nausea, weakness, and weight loss. She appeared pale and wasted and had minimal icterus and a palpable liver. The clinical impression was "metastatic carcinoma, site of origin unknown." Numerous tests and consultations were scheduled, but before they could be carried out, a more discerning physical examination unveiled a smooth tongue and palpable spleen. Pernicious anemia was suspected and proved.

Comment. Some CA is PA.

CASE 4. A sixty-five-year-old man with known systemic hypertension and diabetes mellitus was found on his bathroom floor complaining of chest and back pain. On arrival at the hospital, he was hypotensive and diaphoretic with normal breath sounds and a normal cardiac examination. An electrocardiogram showed sinus rhythm and ST segment elevation in the inferior leads. Chest x-ray demonstrated a tortuous aorta, prominence of the aortic arch, and clear lung fields.

The clinical suspicion was acute inferior myocardial infarction causing cardiogenic shock. Consequently, dopamine and recombinant tissue-type plasminogen activator were administered, but the patient died shortly thereafter. Autopsy showed a dissecting aneurysm of the thoracic aorta but no myocardial infarction.

Comment. This case serves as a sobering reminder that life-saving treatment can be life-threatening if the diagnosis is wrong.

Surely each of us can recall (with regrets) clinical situations in which we were quick to act and slow to think. Perhaps Alexander Pope had us in mind when he wrote, "Fools rush in where angels fear to tread."

Let us not be fools—or fooled. Let us, instead, remember the rattlesnake. If we do, we will always be circumspect with our patients, and they will always get what they deserve—good care.

Selected Reading

Alexander Pope. An essay on criticism. III, 1.66.

Gruver RH, Freis ED. A study of diagnostic errors. Ann Intern Med 47:108, 1957.

Kamp TJ et al. Myocardial infarction, aortic dissection, and thrombolytic therapy. Am Heart J 128:1234, 1994.

Washing Our Hands of the Matter

Plays based on the Bible were popular long before secular acting came into vogue. One of the favorite scenes in those biblical dramas was the enactment of Jesus' trial before Pontius Pilate, the Roman procurator who ordered the crucifixion. To make the action realistic, it was customary to bring in a basin of water. Pilate then washed his hands, disclaiming responsibility for the death sentence. This bit of stage play was a big hit with audiences. As a result, we now speak of "washing our hands of the matter" when we want nothing further to do with a situation.

Washing the hands has another important historical link. A century and a half ago, Ignaz Philipp Semmelweis believed that students performing autopsies on victims of puerperal fever were carrying the infection to healthy mothers in the obstetrical ward. He concluded that washing one's hands before examining women in labor could save lives. Although history ultimately proved him right, obstetricians and midwives of that era vehemently rejected his doctrine of cleanliness. Dispirited and exhausted, Semmelweis finally entered an asylum where he died, ironically, of streptococcal blood poisoning—the very disease he had struggled so hard to prevent.

Today, we know that contaminated hands can transmit pathogens causing respiratory, urinary, enteric, cutaneous, and surgical site infections. We also know that plain soap and running water—when used for at least 10 to 15 seconds—will remove most transiently acquired organisms. Hand washing, therefore, is an integral part of preventing and controlling contagion. Yet, studies continue to show that hospital personnel fail to follow recommended hand-washing practices more than half the time. And physicians are among the worst offenders.

Why is compliance so poor? The main reason is "busyness"—perceived or real. Hence, compliance is lower in intensive care units than elsewhere in the hospital. Other reasons include scarcity of available sinks, skin irritation and dryness resulting from frequent hand washing, and ignorance of the fact that routine patient contact (e.g., measuring the blood pressure or pulse) can contaminate the caregiver's hands.

Health care workers aren't the only ones guilty of bad hand-washing habits. The next time you're in a locker room or public rest room, notice how many people *don't* wash their hands after using the toilet. Some of those individuals carry disease, which they disseminate in various ways, especially by preparing or serving food. But they aren't likely to wash their hands *when* they should until they understand *why* they should. In that light, we in the medical profession can help by spreading the word—and practicing what we preach.

Let's stop "washing our hands of the matter" and start washing our hands of the "matter."

Selected Reading

Boyce JM. It is time for action: Improving hand hygiene in hospitals. Ann Intern Med 130:153, 1999.

Jarvis WR. Handwashing—the Semmelweis lesson forgotten? Lancet 344:1311, 1994.

Larson EL. APIC guideline for handwashing and hand antisepsis in health care settings. Am J Infect Control 23:251, 1995.

Pittet D, Mourouga P, Perneger TV. Compliance with handwashing in a teaching hospital. Ann Intern Med 130:126, 1999.

Sproat LJ, Inglis TJJ. A multicentre survey of hand hygiene practice in intensive care units. J Hosp Infect 26:137, 1994.

Digital Rectal Examination During Early Acute MI*

"Rectal: deferred."

This notation frequently appears in hospital medical charts. In most cases, it means that the physician either forgot to perform a digital rectal examination (DRE) or considered the procedure to be unnecessary, unimportant, or simply inconvenient. But in cases of acute myocardial infarction (AMI), it also signifies this notion: DRE might induce a serious, or even fatal, hemodynamic or rhythm disturbance.

What accounts for the widespread practice of deferring DRE in the early hours of AMI? Some supporting evidence comes from isolated case reports and letters describing untoward effects of DRE. John Kostis, for example, observed ventricular fibrillation during DRE of a man with AMI and recommended that unless DRE is indicated for specific reasons, it should be postponed for two to three weeks. Roy Scott and Salvatore Sancetta could invariably induce Stokes-Adams attacks by gentle rectal stimulation of a woman with complete heart block. And, in carrying out prostate examinations on approximately 2,500 young servicemen, Robert Bilbro observed eight episodes of frank syncope or marked faintness after exerting moderate pressure on the prostate for two to eight seconds. From this, he concluded that AMI is a relative contra-indication to routine rectal examination.

---

* Joseph R. Lee, M.D., is coauthor of this article.

Another concern in performing DRE soon after AMI is the potentially harmful hemodynamic consequences of the Valsalva maneuver, a common accompaniment of DRE. L. J. Klein and coworkers induced syncope in normal volunteers by combining this maneuver with hyperventilation. Similarly, Norman Shaftel and colleagues noted that of 209 healthy adults undergoing the Valsalva maneuver, 47 (22.5 percent) had electrocardiographic changes consistent with mycocardial ischemia. And in a subsequent investigation of ten patients with known angina pectoris, Shaftel's group found that this maneuver intensified the pretest electrocardiographic abnormalities in all ten and caused an anginal attack in six.

The foregoing reports notwithstanding, most studies of rectal stimulation in cardiac patients have shown no adverse effects. In performing rigid sigmoidoscopy on twenty-seven patients with coronary artery disease, Gerald Fletcher and associates observed no catastrophic arrhythmias. Patricia Gruber found that measuring the temperature per rectum in nineteen patients with AMI produced no bradycardias or other arrhythmias. In fact, turning the patient caused a greater increase in heart rate than did taking the temperature rectally. And Carl Pepine and Leslie Wiener reported that even during the Valsalva maneuver, eighteen of twenty-four patients with active angina pectoris actually had *relief* of symptoms and manifested no detrimental hemodynamic or electrocardiographic changes.

Almost thirty years ago, David Earnest and Gerald Fletcher evaluated the safety of a "gentle" rectal examination in eighty-six patients with AMI. They performed the procedure within twenty-four hours of the patient's admission to a cardiac intensive care unit. Although they observed no adverse clinical or electrocardiographic changes, these authors did not say how much time had elapsed between the onset of ischemic pain and performance of DRE. They concluded that patients with myocardial infarction who do not have cardiogenic shock or life-threatening arrhythmias should undergo a rectal examination to detect prostate enlargement, stool impaction, and intestinal bleeding.

We, in turn, have prospectively determined the immediate hemodynamic and electrocardiographic effects of DRE in forty patients with AMI (unpublished data). In most of them, we performed the examination within eight hours of the onset of chest pain (range, 2–19 hours). Before the procedure, we measured the patient's blood pressure and obtained a 12-lead electrocardiogram. During the procedure, and for five minutes thereafter, we monitored a continuous rhythm strip. We recorded the blood pressure during DRE and one and five minutes later. Then we repeated a 12-lead electrocardiogram.

All of our patients had sinus rhythm and normal blood pressure at the time of DRE. No appreciable changes occurred in the heart rate or blood pressure during or after the procedure. Additionally, no changes appeared in the rhythm or electrocardiographic morphology.

Thus, our findings confirm those of Earnest and Fletcher and underscore the fact that if the patient is hemodynamically stable and has no serious arrhythmia, DRE is safe, even during the first two hours after myocardial infarction. Information gained from DRE in such patients can be useful in planning bowel and bladder care and in making decisions regarding anticoagulant and thrombolytic therapy.

In closing, we refer to Joseph Sapira, who, in his magnificent book on bedside diagnosis, emphasized the value of DRE this way: "If you don't put your finger in it, you'll put your foot in it."

Selected Reading

Bilbro RH. Syncope after prostatic examination (letter). N Engl J Med 282:167, 1970.

Earnest DL, Fletcher GF. Danger of rectal examination in patients with acute myocardial infarction: Fact or fiction? N Engl J Med 281:238, 1969.

Fletcher GF et al. Electrocardiographic changes during routine sigmoidoscopy. Arch Intern Med 122:483, 1968.

Gruber PA. Changes in cardiac rate associated with the use of the rectal thermometer in the patient with acute myocardial infarction. Heart Lung 3:288, 1974.

Klein LJ et al. Syncope induced by the Valsalva maneuver: A study of the effects of arterial blood gas tensions, glucose concentration, and blood pressure. Am J Med 37:263, 1964.

Kostis JB. Ventricular fibrillation during rectal examination in a patient with acute myocardial infarction (letter). Chest 72:265, 1977.

Pepine CJ, Wiener L. Effects of the Valsalva maneuver on myocardial ischemia in patients with coronary artery disease. Circulation 59:1304, 1979.

Sapira JD. The rectum: *In* The Art and Science of Bedside Diagnosis, Sapira JD (Ed). Williams & Wilkins, Baltimore, 1990, pp 411–14.

Scott RW, Sancetta SM. Stokes-Adams attacks induced by rectal stimulation in a patient with complete heart block. Circulation 2:886, 1950.

Shaftel N et al. Electrocardiographic changes produced by the Valsalva maneuver in healthy adults. Am J Cardiol 5:473, 1960.

Shaftel N, Shaftel HE, Halpern A. Work-stressor tests and coronary disease. Angiology 13:488, 1962.

The Interesting Patient

"We're sorry, Dr. Fred, but we don't have any interesting patients today."

"And I'm sorry we don't have any interested house officers today."

That brief discourse occasionally takes place when I arrive to conduct teaching rounds. I suspect that medical educators everywhere have similar experiences.

Categorizing patients as interesting—or not interesting—is a habit that all physicians have. It starts in medical school, reaches a peak during postgraduate training, and persists to varying degrees throughout our professional careers. In fact, it becomes so much a part of us that we rarely give it any thought. We should.

Like beauty, the interesting patient is in the eye of the beholder. A woman with argyria, for example, would be interesting to a dermatologist but not necessarily to an orthopedic surgeon. Similarly, a man with a dissecting aneurysm of the aorta would be interesting to a cardiologist but perhaps not to a psychiatrist. And a big liver would be more interesting to a medical student who had never felt one than to a veteran clinician who had felt hundreds. Nevertheless, any patient can be interesting if the doctor is interested.

According to V. Grann (see "The Interesting Patient Syndrome," Arch Intern Med 116:442, 1965), the interesting patient generally has a rare disease (e.g., carcinoid syndrome), an ordinary disease with an atypical pattern (e.g., epilepsy manifesting as abdominal pain), or a pseudodisease—several common but unassociated findings masquerading as a rare disease (e.g., round facies, obesity, hypertension, and diabetes mellitus suggesting Cushing syndrome). He further believes that interesting patients gain extra benefits. They are examined and followed not only by their own physician but by other doctors as well. Moreover, the increased attention enables them to build tremendous ego strength in what otherwise might be a chronic, depressive illness. They become knowledgeable about their disease and can discuss it scientifically with anybody. And they find consolation by uniting with other victims of the same disease to form support groups.

The interesting patient syndrome has its disadvantages, too. Because of the unusual attention interesting patients get, they may try to prolong their illness. They also run the risks of repeated hospitalizations and the discomfort and dangers of numerous tests. And all of these extra activities are expensive.

But the biggest disadvantage of the interesting patient syndrome is the effect it has on most of the people who seek our help—the people with common, everyday illnesses. They are the unfortunate ones whom we wittingly or unwittingly deem "not interesting." As a result, we end up dedicating our best efforts to the few rather than to the many. We also lose a great opportunity to educate ourselves, because every patient—interesting or not—is a challenge and can teach us something.

Now ask yourself these questions: How would *you* feel if you were the patient and your doctor deemed your problem uninteresting? Would you agree? Would you understand? Would you forgive? Would you return?

Incidentally, how many interesting *doctors* do you know?

Algorithms: Let's Give Them Back

Ever since my residency training in the mid-1950s, I have made a habit of reading at least one medical article every day. That habit has not only kept me informed but also enabled me to appreciate ongoing changes in the content and format of medical writings. I have noticed, for example, that abstracts at the front of articles have largely replaced summaries at the end of articles. And with the burgeoning advances in medical technology, detailed clinical descriptions have all but disappeared, and a lopsided emphasis on laboratory data has emerged.

Something else has crept into the medical literature with little fanfare but with increasing frequency and popularity—the algorithm.

The American Heritage Dictionary of the English Language defines algorithm as "any mechanical or recursive occupational procedure." Wondering exactly what recursive meant, I returned to the dictionary and learned that recursive is the adjectival form of recursion, which is "a mathematical expression, such as a polynomial, each term of which is determined by application of a formula to preceding terms." Befuddled by these definitions, I opened *Mrs. Byrne's Dictionary of Unusual, Obscure, and Preposterous Words.* At "algorithm," it offered me only "a rule of procedure for solving recurrent mathematical problems." In desperation, I consulted *Dorland's Illustrated Medical Dictionary.* It calls an algorithm "a step-by-step method of solving a problem or making decisions, as in making a diagnosis; an established mechanical procedure for solving certain mathematical problems."

From these various sources, I concluded that an algorithm is a tool that physicians have borrowed from mathematicians to solve diagnostic (and sometimes therapeutic) problems. Therein lies my first objection to the use of algorithms in medical practice. Mathematicians manage numbers. Physicians manage patients. Sadly, however, more and more physicians are managing numbers rather than the patients who have those numbers. And algorithms undoubtedly contribute to this deplorable trend.

Another drawback of algorithms is their all-too-frequent complexity. On occasion, I see algorithms that occupy an entire printed page. They have so many steps with so many arrows pointing in so many directions that I ultimately give up trying to figure everything out.

Do algorithms need to be so complicated? I think not. But I do think that some journal editors, as well as some authors and publishers, opt for bulk over brevity, size over substance, matter over mind. Furthermore, padding and puffery ostensibly make the algorithm appear more "scholarly," thereby increasing its chances for publication.

Do algorithms leave room for clinical judgment and compassion? No. Incorporating these requisite qualities into a purely mechanical procedure is clearly impossible.

Do algorithms take into account the wide variation in disease manifestations and in patient responses? Certainly not. By their inanimate nature, algorithms cannot compensate for animate variations.

Do algorithms improve the patient-doctor relationship? No, they replace it—the doctor interacts with the algorithm, not the patient.

Do algorithms reduce costs? Some physicians say yes. I say no. Studies have shown that a carefully obtained medical history, coupled with a good physical examination and a bit of thought, can make the diagnosis in up to 90 percent of cases. This time-honored approach is unquestionably cheaper and less time-consuming than mindlessly following a maze of mechanical steps that often involve expensive investigations.

Do algorithms enhance patient care? Again, some physicians believe they do, but I disagree. Look at it this way. Algorithms in medicine are much like cookbooks. They furnish recipes for the novice. As with fine chefs, however, well-informed and well-trained physicians don't need them and commonly ignore them. And as all of us know, recipes in the hands of the novice don't produce haute cuisine.

I'm not the only one who thinks this way. In a discussion of clinical problem-solving, Jerome P. Kassirer, former Editor-in-Chief of *The New England Journal of Medicine,* said this about algorithms: "In recent years several new diagnostic approaches have been introduced. Algorithms and practice guidelines codify the sequential steps the clinician should take in 'working up' a patient. Unfortunately, elaborate and rigid flowcharts cannot be expected to yield the correct diagnosis regularly or to substitute for the careful probing of a skilled diagnostician who uses an iterative process—gathering and interpreting information and revising hypotheses—until a diagnosis is reached."

So for the reasons cited, I suggest that we give algorithms back to the mathematicians—and focus instead on expanding our medical knowledge, honing our bedside skills, strengthening our clinical judgment, and displaying compassion. If we do, our patients will be the better for it.

Selected Reading

Cutler P. Problem Solving in Clinical Medicine: From Data to Diagnosis, 3rd edn. Williams & Wilkins, Baltimore, 1998, p 33.

Kassirer JP. Teaching problem-solving: How are we doing? N Engl J Med 332:1507, 1995.

Sackett DL et al. Clinical Epidemiology: A Basic Science for Clinical Medicine, 2nd edn. Little, Brown and Company, Boston, 1991, pp 8–12, 95, 298–99, 326.
Sapira JD. The Art and Science of Bedside Diagnosis. Urban & Schwartzenberg, Baltimore, 1990, p 33.

The Numbers Game

It is a silly game where nobody wins.
–*Gnomologia* by Thomas Fuller (1654–1734),
English physician and writer of maxims

A serious malady pervades and undermines our profession. I call it the numbers game—treating a number (or some test result) rather than the patient who has that number. The following cases illustrate the physical, financial, and emotional price that patients pay when physicians play this game.

CASE 1. A seventy-two-year-old woman complained of weakness and progressive weight loss of five months' duration. The cause turned out to be apathetic (masked) hyperthyroidism. Her physician planned to treat her with radioactive iodine, but opted for thyroidectomy when he learned that she had a history of possible allergy to iodine-containing contrast material.

The patient's preoperative hemoglobin concentration was 9.8 g/dL, but the anesthesiologist would not put her to sleep until it was at least 10 g/dL. Consequently, she received two units of packed red blood cells. Unfortunately, she got the wrong blood and had a severe transfusion reaction that left her brain-dead. Shortly thereafter, she died.

Comment. Treating a hemoglobin "deficit" of 0.2 g/dL cost this patient her life. Had her physician simply repeated the hemoglobin determination, the tragedy might have been averted. Moreover, the anesthesiologist's widely held notion—that a favorable anesthetic outcome requires a preoperative hemoglobin concentration of 10 g/dL or greater—has little scientific support. Indeed, strong evidence to the contrary is readily available. And her physician should have known that an allergy to *organic* iodine does not preclude the therapeutic use of radioactive *inorganic* iodine.

CASE 2. A sixty-nine-year-old woman was admitted to the surgical service for management of acute cholecystitis. Her initial blood pressure as determined by a nurse was 135/80 mm Hg. With symptomatic care only, her condition remained stable until the third hospital day, when a different nurse found the patient's blood pressure to be 70/40 mm Hg. This finding prompted transfer of the patient to the intensive care unit with a presumptive diagnosis of sepsis.

For the next two days, she received antibiotics intravenously and was seen by a staff surgeon, cardiologist, pulmonologist, and critical care physician. Her blood pressure recordings during that time ranged from 135/80 to 140/90 mm Hg. No cause for the "hypotension" emerged, so she was transferred to the medical service for further observation.

Two days later, a nurse reported that the patient's blood pressure was again 70/40 mm Hg. Because the patient did not appear to be ill, her physicians decided to examine her more carefully. They discovered that her right radial pulse was strong and that her blood pressure in that arm was 135/80 mm Hg. In her left arm, however, the radial pulse was barely palpable and the blood pressure was 70/40 mm Hg. A magnetic resonance angiogram demonstrated stenosis of the left subclavian artery.

But the numbers game was not over. In preparation for cholecystectomy, the patient was sent to the cardiac laboratory for a stress test. Soon after she arrived, a cardiac fellow who was new on the case placed a frantic call to her internist informing him that the patient's blood pressure was 70/40 mm Hg. Fortunately, the game ended there.

Comment. This woman would have been better off had she been hospitalized thirty to fifty years ago. In those days, physicians routinely checked the pulses in all four extremities and measured the blood pressure in both arms. Nowadays they do not. In fact, many, if not most, of them do not even take the blood pressure themselves. They simply accept the measurement taken by a nurse or some other assistant and treat the patient accordingly.

A variety of specialists and subspecialists saw this patient on numerous occasions over a six-day span before they finally examined her properly. Treating her numbers without regard for her total clinical picture unduly extended her hospital stay, needlessly prompted her transfer to the intensive care unit, and clearly gouged a big hole in her pocketbook.

CASE 3. A fifteen-year-old girl sought medical attention for a red, bumpy, and sometimes itchy rash on her face and arms. The rash would appear after prolonged exposure to sunlight and would slowly fade in a few days. She had no other complaints. Her physician ordered an antinuclear antibody (ANA) test, and when it came back positive, he told her that she probably had an early connective tissue disease, most likely systemic lupus erythematosus (SLE).

The though of having SLE devastated her. A close friend in high school had died of SLE, and fear of the same fate remained uppermost in the patient's mind. For the next thirteen years, she took no medications and remained physically well. She never had joint pain, Raynaud's phenomenon, hair loss, dryness of the eyes or mouth, oral ulcers, pleurisy, or unexplained gastrointestinal or genitourinary symptoms. But she refused to get married, thinking that she would be a burden to her husband and children.

Because of a promising job offer, she moved to another state and presented to a rheumatologist for follow-up care. Review of her accompanying medical records showed that over the years, her complete blood counts, serum creatinine values, liver function tests, urinalyses, and serum complement levels had been normal; her ANA titers had ranged from 1/640 to 1/320 in a homogeneous or speckled pattern; and antibodies to DNA, ribonucleoprotein, and hepatitis virus had been absent. Biopsy of a skin lesion had shown "spongiotic dermatitis without evidence of SLE."

The rheumatologist told the patient that she had no evidence of SLE or any other connective tissue disease. He discussed with her the many causes of a positive ANA test in a young woman and offered her various ways to protect against the sun's rays. She then broke into tears, expressed immense relief at not having a chronic illness, and said she felt as though her life had been given back to her.

Comment. This case exemplifies the all-too-frequent misinterpretation of an elevated ANA titer. Numerous studies have shown that ANA test results may be positive not only in SLE but also in other rheumatic diseases, in a wide variety of nonrheumatic diseases, and in 3 percent to 30 percent of healthy people. Failure of the physician to appreciate these facts created long-standing emotional turmoil for this patient.

The High-tech Addiction

The numbers game in medicine has been around a long time. However, its popularity has skyrocketed in recent years. I believe that this accelerated popularity results primarily from the addictive nature of modern technology. With so many sophisticated tests and procedures at our disposal, we have fallen in love with numbers and have unwittingly acquired a laboratory-oriented rather than a patient-oriented mind-set. Inadequate training, insufficient clinical experience, and plain old ignorance undoubtedly contribute to this behavior. Yet, board-certified private practitioners and faculty members of two medical schools were active participants in the cases presented here.

And let us not overlook the shackles of managed care. Health maintenance organizations have forced physicians to care for a maximum *number* of patients in a minimal *number* of minutes for the lowest *number* of dollars.

Can we slow down or stop this numbers game? Only if we concentrate on taking good medical histories, doing careful physical examinations, and then thinking about our patients. Only if we are willing to be role models of honesty and integrity for each other. And only if we constantly remember that the practice of medicine is a calling, not a game.

Selected Reading

Corwin HL. Blood transfusion: First, do no harm! Chest 116:1149, 1999.

Goodnough LT et al. Transfusion medicine—blood transfusion. N Engl J Med 340:438, 1999.

Illei GG, Klippel JH. Why is the ANA result positive? Bull Rheum Dis 48 (January): 1, 1999.

Jeffares AN, Gray M. A Dictionary of Quotations. Barnes and Noble Books, New York, 1995, p 270.

Moder KG. Use and interpretation of rheumatologic tests: A guide for clinicians. Mayo Clin Proc 71:391, 1996.

Richardson B, Epstein WV. Utility of the fluorescent antinuclear antibody test in a single patient. Ann Intern Med 95:333, 1981.

Welch HG, Meehan KR, Goodnough LT. Prudent strategies for elective red blood cell transfusion. Ann Intern Med 116:393, 1992.

ON SCHOOLING THE PHYSICIAN

For us oldies in medicine, doing nothing means doing a lot. It means not ordering expensive, state-of-the-art studies when cheaper, conventional tests would supply the same information. It means not administering a slew of medications in an attempt to alleviate every possible ill. It means not requesting numerous consultations just because the diagnosis is not immediately obvious. It means appreciating the opportunities to learn the natural history of disease. It means realizing that many patients get well in spite of what we do, not because of what we do.

–H. L. F. in "Doing Nothing"

Maxwell Wintrobe once wrote, "…many look, but few see." Today, few see because few look.

–H. L. F. in "Requiem for the Ophthalmoscope"

Doing Nothing

An harassed merchant went to his rabbi and complained. "I'm in terrible trouble. I can't support my wife and seven children, and every year there comes still another baby. What should I do?"

The wise old rabbi thought for a moment, then responded: "Don't do anything!"

–Anonymous

Hurrah for the rabbi! When faced with the merchant's plight, he didn't scurry to consult other rabbis. He didn't call in a banker to finance a loan. He didn't seek social services or foster homes for the seven children. Instead, he took time to think about the matter; and the solution he offered illustrates an important point—doing nothing can be the best way to handle a problem.

Centuries ago, the poet John Milton emphasized the value of doing nothing. "They also serve who only stand and wait,"[1] he wrote. In the mid-1950s, when I was in residency training, my mentors continually hammered home this point. As late as the mid-1970s, doing nothing still had its proponents: "The well trained doctor knows what to do for his patient; the especially well trained doctor knows what not to do."[2] Since then, this approach has received little attention in the classroom, at the bedside, or in the medical literature. Consequently, the art of doing nothing has become almost extinct.

For us oldies in medicine, doing nothing means doing a lot. It means not ordering expensive, state-of-the-art studies when cheaper, conventional tests would supply the same information. It means not administering a slew of medications in an attempt to alleviate every possible ill. It means not requesting numerous consultations just because the diagnosis is not immediately obvious. It means appreciating the opportunities to learn the natural history of disease. It means realizing that many patients get well in spite of what we do, not because of what we do.

Today's medical students, house officers, and young practitioners cannot fathom doing nothing. The reasons seem clear. They lack the necessary role models. They get taught to rely on sophisticated machinery and superspecialists, not on their minds and five senses. They know that insurance companies and federal agencies don't pay for thinking, for observing patients closely, or for other types of disciplined inaction. They know that disciplined inaction invites pressure from their peers, dissatisfaction from their patients, and criticism from their teachers. They fear that such inaction will trigger court action. They end up prisoners of the system, shackled to routine. No wonder they have a "nothing doing" attitude toward "doing nothing."

With that attitude, they will never learn how and when to do nothing. And their patients will pay for that ignorance.

References

[1] Milton, John. On His Blindness. London, 1652.

[2] Hardy HL. Annual discourse—risk and responsibility. A physician's viewpoint. N Engl J Med 293:801–806, 1975.

Previous Medical Records: Lest We Forget

Information from previous medical records can be crucial, both to patient care and to physician education. Yet, on teaching rounds these days, I find that such records get little more than lip service. House officers frequently don't try to obtain them, rarely appreciate the need to get them promptly, and generally show limited ability to scrutinize them effectively once in hand. And these records typically are missing at case presentations.

The genesis of this problem seems clear: Medicine has moved from "high touch" to "high tech," and medical education has shifted its focus accordingly. As a consequence, today's trainees, many of their teachers, and many private practitioners are becoming prisoners of the laboratory, deprived of the joy and satisfaction of using one's mind and five senses to make diagnoses. Thus, they often overlook an integral part of the medical history—the patient's medical records.

The following cases, all from major teaching hospitals, illustrate what happens when house officers and attending physicians alike fail to take advantage of previous medical records.

Lung Mass in a Smoker

An asymptomatic fifty-seven-year-old man with a long history of smoking had a routine chest x-ray that showed an irregular 2 × 2-cm mass in the right lower lobe. Five years earlier, he had undergone treatment at another hospital for what he said was pneumonia. His physicians now suspected lung cancer and ordered cytologic examination of the sputum; the results were negative.

Consultation with a pulmonologist led to bronchoscopy and transbronchial biopsy, neither of which disclosed an abnormality. Thoracotomy then revealed an old pulmonary infarct.

Comment. Previous chest films should always be reviewed before submitting a patient to exploratory thoracotomy. In this case, the physicians did not question the patient's history of pneumonia or wonder whether that illness might have been related to the present findings. Consequently, they did not examine the available records or previous chest x-rays from the other hospital. Had they done so, they would have found a discharge diagnosis of pulmonary infarction and a discharge chest x-ray identical to the current one. Their oversight cost the patient part of his lung and a lot of his money.

Back Pain and an Abdominal Mass

An eighty-five-year-old woman presented with progressive back pain of several weeks' duration. She said that she had had a renal cancer removed two and a half years earlier.

Physical examination demonstrated a palpable abdominal mass that her physician thought was an aortic aneurysm. Abdominal sonography confirmed a mass, but aortography was normal. Films of the thoracic and lumbar spine disclosed compression fractures of T-12 and L-1. MRI suggested neoplasm as the cause of the collapsed vertebrae. Fine-needle aspiration of T-12 proved inconclusive, but open biopsy of this vertebra demonstrated carcinoma consistent with a renal cell origin. The patient then received palliative radiation therapy to her spine.

Subsequently, this case was reviewed at a tumor conference. Examination of the patient's previous medical records uncovered some disquieting facts. At nephrectomy—done in the same hospital—the tumor had already spread to multiple paraaortic lymph nodes.

Furthermore, an abdominal CT scan done six months before the admission for back pain had shown a mass, strongly suggestive of metastatic disease, engulfing the midportions of the aorta and vena cava.

Comment. It is difficult to understand or excuse the attending physician's failure to obtain this patient's medical records, especially when he knew that she had undergone a nephrectomy for renal cancer just two and a half years earlier. Had he known the information in those records, he would not have pursued the possibility of an abdominal aortic aneurysm, nor would he necessarily have biopsied the patient's spine. And the patient, in turn, would have been spared the expense of hospitalization, the discomfort and risks of aortography and open vertebral biopsy, and the delay in starting her palliative radiation therapy.

Hematologic Complications After Lumbar Surgery

A seventy-nine-year-old man entered the hospital for evaluation of chronic low back pain and leg numbness. Two previous lumbar disk operations had afforded him no relief.

Physical examination was unremarkable except for areflexia in the lower extremities. The hemoglobin was 10.8, total leukocyte count 20,000, and platelet count 110,000. A peripheral blood film showed occasional myelocytes and metamyelocytes. A CT scan and MRI of the lumbar spine and lumbar myelography demonstrated severe spinal stenosis.

The patient underwent lumbar spinal surgery. The procedure involved a standard posterior incision, a laparotomy for anterior exposure of the vertebrae, and the placement of extensive supportive hardware. During the operation, he bled profusely, necessitating transfusions with plasma, platelets, packed cells, and autologous salvaged blood.

Postoperatively, the total leukocyte count rose to 100,000, prompting hematologic consultation. The patient's wife told the consultant that two years earlier her husband had been diagnosed as having chronic granulocytic leukemia. Medical records obtained from their hometown verified her story. They also indicated that the patient's platelet count had been falling gradually, and that he recently had gone to an emergency room because of an uncontrollable nosebleed.

That important information came too late. The patient required two more trips to the operating room—one for evacuation of blood clots and control of oozing from incision sites, the other for removal of infected hardware. After three months of hospitalization, he died.

Comment. Results of this patient's admission blood studies should have prompted hematologic evaluation *preoperatively.* Had that taken place, or had the patient's medical history been documented more carefully from the outset, he might have been managed differently, and might still be alive.

Fatigue, Edema, and Anemia

A fifty-year-old rancher entered the hospital for workup of anemia. He was asymptomatic except for fatigue. On physical examination, the only abnormality was symmetric edema of the feet and lower legs. His hematocrit was 31 percent, and the red cells were normochromic and normocytic. Other routine laboratory tests, including a chest x-ray and electrocardiogram, were normal. Extensive studies during ten days of hospitalization failed to uncover the cause of the anemia, and the patient went home—undiagnosed and untreated.

One month later, he returned to the hospital with the same findings—fatigue, swollen legs, and anemia. Numerous investigations again failed to establish the cause. At this point, the hematology fellow collected all of the accumulated data and made an important discovery: During the first hospitalization, the patient's peripheral edema had resolved and the hematocrit had risen to 42 percent, both spontaneously.

Next, he compared the admission and discharge chest x-rays. To his surprise, the heart size, although normal initially, had become distinctly smaller before discharge. He then compared the discharge x-ray with the one taken at the second admission. The finding was predictable—the heart had "enlarged" in the interim.

The puzzle was solved—dilutional anemia resulting from congestive heart failure. After therapy with diuretics and digitalis, the anemia and edema rapidly resolved, and the heart again returned to its small size.

Comment: Hurrah for the hematology fellow! He reviewed *all* of the available evidence, not just the discharge summary or portions of the written record. By retrieving and examining the chest films himself, he found the key to the puzzle—changing heart size. Even so, had he done his sleuthing earlier, he could have shortened the second hospitalization.

Conclusion

These four cases exemplify what James B. Herrick warned against almost seventy years ago. In discussing the training of clinicians, he said:

> There is a tendency…to overestimate the value of the instrumental and the laboratory side of clinical medicine. There is an air of finality about these tests that is far from warranted by the facts, but it attracts us. To elicit a history or to make a physical examination is commonly looked on as not very scientific.… We all recognize that such teaching or practice is wrong. It trains the student not to examine or to think but to resort to a test tube, a mechanical device or the knife of the surgeon. Worst of all, the student or prac-

> titioner does not think even when the results of these tests come in to him. He lets someone else do the interpreting. He accepts a long distance finding at its face value. He forgets the possibility of error on the part of the method or the technician.... If we were to analyze our failures in diagnosis, we should find that they depended more on a hasty or incomplete history or the loose interpretation of the history than on careless or slovenly physical examination or neglected special test.

Today, in the era of high-tech medicine, we need to remember the value of a carefully documented medical history, which includes attention to previous medical records. If we forget, cases like those described here will only increase in number. And the consequences will be costly—more ill-advised procedures, higher medical bills, and greater patient suffering.

Selected Reading

Herrick JB. The clinician of the future. JAMA 86:1, 1926.

The Blind Leading the Blind

The deflection of faculty attention away from medical students occurred in the clinical departments. There, much of the responsibility for teaching came to be exercised by house officers. Students saw their attending physicians regularly, but it was the residents and interns whom they saw on a moment-to-moment basis. For students, the quality of a clerkship depended as much on the resident as it did on the faculty attending. A good resident had the power to create a sense of belonging so that the student felt like a true member of the ward team. An insensitive or disdainful resident who provided "scut work" and ridicule instead of teaching and encouragement was a student's mightmare. With difficult residents, students had little choice but to endure, knowing the rotation would end and hoping that in the next they might be more fortunate. If students were lucky, they could learn from these negative examples. If not, they could be scarred for life. (p. 74)

As house officers could enrich or ruin a student's clinical clerkship, students could similarly affect a house officer's experience. (p. 97)

By 1960, 56 percent of faculty time at the school was devoted to research, while only 14 percent was spent on undergraduate medical education. (p. 215)

> Any doubt that teaching was subordinate to research could be laid to rest by examining the reward system of medical schools. Everywhere, promotion and academic advancement resulted mainly from research... [A]t some schools being known as a good teacher could even be "an obstacle to advancement." (p. 216)
>
> [T]hese observations are to suggest that good teaching in the modern medical school...was frequently by accident rather than by design. (p. 218)

Those excerpts are from a new 514-page book that has been nominated for a Pulitzer prize in nonfiction. It is *Time to Heal: American Medical Education from the Turn of the Century to the Era of Managed Care* (Oxford University Press, New York, 1999) by Kenneth M. Ludmerer, Professor of Medicine in the School of Medicine and Professor of History on the Faculty of Arts and Sciences at Washington University, St. Louis. Prominent medical educators, historians, and editors are hailing this book as the most scholarly, comprehensive, and meticulously referenced report dealing with medical education in the twentieth century. In my view, it is must reading, not only for everyone involved in medical education but also for anyone interested in the turmoil that currently engulfs health care.

The Problem

The excerpts brilliantly elucidate the fact that American medical schools value research over teaching. This stance had little detrimental effect on medical education for most of the past century. But now, with the ever-increasing emphasis on technology, shrinking government funding of medical services, and the devastating impact of managed care, clinical teaching has suffered a serious blow. Medical schools are so strapped for money these days that they force the clinical faculty to spend more and more time caring for paying patients and less and less time caring for medical students and house officers. As a result, trainees are left to fend for themselves in the quest for competency, unaware of how much better their lot could and should be.

At present, house officers learn clinical medicine primarily from each other rather than from veteran clinicians. Students, in turn, learn clinical medicine primarily from house officers who are only several years their senior and not necessarily more knowledgeable or competent. This arrangement had merit many years ago when residencies, in contrast to internships, were reserved for the elite. In those days, acceptance into a residency provided no guarantee of completing it. And since most training programs had a pyramid structure, attrition always occurred, with only the best residents remaining. From that group, one resident ultimately became the chief resident, who also served as assistant to the department chair.

Today, residency positions are much more numerous and easier to obtain. And with the pyramid structure largely a relic of the past, the relative number of weak residents has risen. In many ways, therefore, we now have a see-one, do-one, teach-one system—a system that fosters mediocrity, stifles individuality, promotes incompetence, and permits, if not encourages, dishonesty.

Illustrative Cases

CASE 1. On teaching rounds recently, a second-year medical resident claimed that his patient had hepatosplenomegaly, but the attending physician disagreed. It turned out that the resident was feeling the patient's ribs, mistaking them for a palpable liver and spleen.

Had this resident's error not been discovered early, the patient probably would have undergone unnecessary and potentially harmful procedures in a fruitless attempt to find a nonexistent disease. And let us not forget that this resident was the ward team's leader who supervised the student and intern on the case.

CASE 2. Last year, a third-year medical resident presented to me the case of a forty-two-year-old *white* man with epigastric pain. When I saw the patient, however, he was obviously a light-skinned *black* man, a fact that the patient promptly verified.

This case, the previous case, and numerous others equally bad are sobering reminders that the course in physical diagnosis at most American medical schools today is woefully inadequate. Many of these courses consist mainly, if not totally, of lectures. And if any hands-on teaching occurs, house officers (even at times senior students or nurses) typically do it.

CASE 3. On reading the medical inpatient record of a sixty-five-year-old man with severe angina pectoris, I noticed that under "Physical Examination," the student, intern, and resident all had written PERRLA (pupils equal, round, and react to light and accommodation). When I asked them whether they actually checked the patient's pupils, each answered, "No." Why, then, did they record it as having been done? "Because it's routine," they said.

Over the years, I have uncovered countless other cases in which students and house officers write PERRLA but never examine the pupils. I also frequently see "cranial nerves intact" when, in fact, cranial nerves I, II, and VIII have not been tested. No matter how you look at it, this seemingly innocuous but common practice is both dishonest and potentially harmful.

CASE 4. A thirty-four-year-old woman was admitted to the hospital because of renal failure. On careful review of her inpatient record, I detected an all-too-frequent phenomenon—the admission write-ups and progress notes by the student, intern, and resident were almost identical. When I questioned them about it, they admitted copying each other's work. Too much to do and too little time to do it was their excuse.

Copycatting may serve some students and house officers, but it never serves the patient.

Fixing This Mess

If you think that I am nitpicking or exaggerating, or that my concerns reflect a local aberration, please think again. I have found the same problems during visits to other medical schools, and colleagues from all parts of the United States assure me that the situation is identical at their institutions.

Fixing this mess will not be easy. Nothing substantive will change until we change our system of health care delivery. That system, as Ludmerer points out, is "forcing physicians to churn through patients in assembly-line fashion at ever-accelerating rates" (p. 384).

The key will be finding ways to slow down that hectic pace. Doing so, however, will require strong professional leadership with solid public support. Once we achieve that goal, doctors will have more time to render good patient care, clinical faculties will have more time to teach, and medical students and house officers will have better opportunities to learn clinical skills.

Then, perhaps, medical schools will shift their focus and get back to the serious business of producing competent physicians. And *until* then, "if the blind lead the blind, both shall fall into the ditch" (Matthew 15:14).

Requiem for the Ophthalmoscope

During a recent morning report at a public hospital, a third-year medical resident presented the case of a forty-six-year-old woman with hemiparesis of sudden onset. When I asked him what he had seen in her eyegrounds, he said, "I didn't look."

Spurred by his response, I led the group to the patient's bedside, intent on examining her optic fundi. But when I asked for an ophthalmoscope, none of the six residents in attendance and none of the interns and students working nearby could accommodate me. What's going on here, I wondered?

My curiosity aroused, I promptly retrieved ten charts from the nurses' station to determine how many write-ups mentioned the optic fundi. Although every chart had entries by a student, intern, and resident, only two made reference to a funduscopic examination. When asked to explain this deficiency, several house officers claimed that their ophthalmoscopes had been stolen. Others considered ophthalmoscopes too bulky to carry in their pockets. The real reason, however, was obvious: Their teachers, including me, had dropped the ball.

I then decided to examine the charts of patients on the internal medicine teaching services of a private hospital and a university hospital. Both facilities have ophthalmoscopes at nurses' stations or in examining rooms, or both. So thievery and accessibility are not factors. At the private hospital, just one of twenty-two randomly selected charts contained a description of the optic fundi. The score at the university hospital was not much better—four of thirty charts.

Having surveyed the academic scene, I turned my attention to private practice. On reviewing at random the records of 27 patients recently discharged from the medicine service of a 200-bed, nonteaching acute care facility, I found descriptions of the optic fundi in *none.* The thirteen physicians of record in these cases were a mixture of general internists, medical subspecialists, and family practitioners. Furthermore, several prominent ophthalmologists who consult in both teaching and nonteaching hospitals told me that referring physicians—regardless of specialty—rarely dilate the pupils or examine the optic fundi before requesting consultation.

Did the results of my investigation represent a local aberration, or did they, as I suspected, typify a national trend? For an answer, I contacted professors in the departments of internal medicine at two distant medical schools—one on the West Coast, the other in the Midwest. One professor confirmed the same shortcoming at his school. The other emphasized that the situation is similar—if not worse—at his center and everywhere he travels.

In a cogent study from the East Coast published eighteen years ago, Stanley Wiener and Morton Nathanson evaluated the performance of physical examination by house staff. Among errors of omission, failure to inspect the retina was frequent with each new group of house officers entering their institution. They observed similar errors when visiting other teaching hospitals in the United States. The problem, therefore, is not new, but it *is* widespread and likely to grow.

And medical schools are not helping the matter. Courses in physical diagnosis, for example, are frequently disjointed, inserted piecemeal into already crowded curricula, and taught by residents, fellows, and junior faculty members. One medical resident told me that in his physical diagnosis course, the only exposure he had to the optic fundus was a lecture by an ophthalmologist who showed slides but gave no hands-on instruction. Other residents told me that during their third and fourth years in medical school, there was no organized attempt to help them acquire skills in using the ophthalmoscope. No wonder they use it so sparingly now.

Why this lament? Because ophthalmoscopy is the only clinical maneuver that allows direct inspection of blood columns and neural structure in vivo. Because it provides at times the first evidence of glaucoma, diabetes mellitus, intracranial hypertension, cholesterol embolization, hyperlipemia, and a host of hematologic, infectious, and vascular diseases. And because making diagnoses in such a safe, quick, and inexpensive manner is gratifying and fun. Furthermore, even after the diagnosis has been made, ophthalmoscopic signs can be particularly useful in assessing the severity, chronicity, and prognosis of the disease.

Maxwell Wintrobe once wrote, "...many look, but few see." Today, few see because few look.

Selected Reading

Wiener S, Nathanson M. Physical examination: Frequently observed errors. JAMA 236:852, 1976.

Greenberger NJ. Whither the patient history and physical examination? Am Coll Phys Dig 10:2, 1990.

Sapira JD. An internist looks at the fundus oculi. Dis Mon 30:1, 1984.

Wintrobe MM. Blood, Pure and Eloquent. McGraw-Hill, New York, 1980, p 720.

Night Sweats

Quickly now: *What's the first thing you think of when a patient has night sweats?*

I recently put that question to a group of medical students, house officers, and senior clinicians (infectious disease specialists, pulmonologists, rheumatologists, oncologists, and generalists). Most said tuberculosis. A few said lymphoma, and one said too many bed covers. On further questioning, all of the clinicians agreed that in their experience, night sweats are neither characteristic of nor common in tuberculosis. Why, then, was tuberculosis the dominant answer? Traditional teaching, I believe.

As far back as the second century A.D., Aretaeus of Cappadocia noted "evening fever sweats" as an accompaniment of what would later be recognized as tuberculosis. Similarly, at the turn of this century, William Osler wrote, "Drenching perspirations are common in phthisis and constitute one of the most distressing features of the disease." In 1951, however, Robert Coope's book on chest diseases offered this observation: "Night sweats [in tuberculosis] have become infinitely less common since the importance of proper hygienic management, sensible clothing, fresh air, and free ventilation has been appreciated." The same year, Harrison's textbook of medicine stated, "Night sweats are considered classic manifestations of tuberculosis, but actually do not occur in most instances until the disease is fairly far advanced." Current texts on internal medicine, pulmonology, and infectious diseases continue to mention night sweats in association with tuberculosis, but few link night sweats with other disorders except lymphoma and Hodgkin's disease.

In a unique study of night sweats published eight years ago, Michele Lea and Robert Aber interviewed 174 patients selected at random from the medicine, surgery, obstetric, and gynecology services of a university hospital. Seventy-two (41 percent) of the patients reported night sweats within the three months before admission. One fourth of the patients also had day sweats.

Night sweats were mild in half of the patients (patient removed bed covers, but no bathing or change of clothing was required), moderate in a quarter (patient arose to wash face or other affected body areas), and severe in the remainder (patient needed bath or change of clothing). Severe sweats were significantly associated with use of antipyretics and were most common in patients on the medicine service. The night sweats were generalized in about half of the patients and localized to a particular area in the rest. Only a fourth of the patients had accompanying fever or chills. Duration of night sweats ranged from one day to twenty-seven years; frequency ranged from nightly to once every two weeks. Obstetric patients had night sweats almost twice as often as did the other patients. Five patients had lymphoma or leukemia. *None had tuberculosis.*

Nocturnal sweating occurs commonly in healthy people who sleep with too much covering or in poorly ventilated rooms under hot, humid conditions. But night sweats can also be a manifestation of hyperthyroidism, endocarditis, temporal arteritis, diabetes mellitus, hypoglycemia, pheochromocytoma, carcinoid syndrome, dysautonomic states, Prinzmetal's angina, diabetes insipidus, solid neoplasms, rheumatic disorders, fungal infections, hypothalamic lesions, anxiety, substance abuse, and use of medications (especially salicylates and acetaminophen).

Despite current knowledge, many patients still undergo tests for tuberculosis just because they have night sweats. We can no longer afford this malady of practice. We should put to rest the long-ingrained notion that night sweats signify tuberculosis.

Selected Reading

Lea MJ, Aber RC. Descriptive epidemiology of night sweats upon admission to a university hospital. South Med J 78:1065, 1985.

Raff SB, Gershberg H. Night sweats: A dominant symptom in diabetes insipidus. JAMA 234:1252, 1975.

To Be *B* or Not to Be *B*: Is That the Question?*

The good doctor, whether general practitioner or specialist, ... studies the patient's personality as well as his disease.[1]
–Sir Hugh Cairns (1896–1952)

The eminent Scottish surgeon, John Hunter (1728–1793), suffered from angina pectoris. He also suffered from a short fuse. One day, immediately following an intensely heated board meeting, Hunter stormed out of the room, collapsed, and died in the arms of a colleague.[2] His case brought to light the powerful influence of emotions on the heart.

Hunter very likely had what modern physicians would call Type A personality, which is characterized by intense ambition, strong competitiveness, and a constant preoccupation with deadlines. Persons lacking these traits are said to have Type B personality. From the cardiac standpoint, the difference between the two types may be important—or it may not.

More than forty years ago, Friedman and Rosenman reported that people with a Type A personality had a seven-fold greater incidence of clinical coronary artery disease than did those with a Type B personality.[3] Since then, many conflicting reports have appeared concerning the relationship between Type A personality and the development and progression of coronary artery disease.[4-7]

---

* Ramesh Hariharan, M.D., is coauthor of this article.

A panel sponsored by the National Institutes of Health in 1981 concluded that Type A behavior constituted an independent risk factor for coronary artery disease.[5] The risk was similar in magnitude to that created by smoking, hypercholesterolemia, or elevated blood pressure. Four years later, however, members of the Multicenter Post-Infarction Research Group argued that there was no uniform evidence to substantiate either a close relation between the characteristic behavior of the Type A personality and coronary artery disease or the protective effects of the Type B personality."[6]

The controversy escalated in 1993, when Lachar suggested that coronary-prone behavior and Type A behavior are not synonymous, and that the coronary-prone patient should not be envisaged as the "achievement-oriented, overburdened workaholic.[8] Instead, coronary-prone behavior appears to include physiologic and emotional reactivity to challenging situations," especially those triggering anger, cynicism, mistrust, and hostility.[8]

Subsequent investigations complicated this issue further. A case-control study of 340 patients by O'Connor and coworkers in 1995 raised the possibility that decreased levels of HDL cholesterol account for the increased risk of nonfatal myocardial infarction in persons with Type A personality.[9] Unfortunately, most other studies on psychosocial risk factors for myocardial infarction have not included data on HDL cholesterol. Consequently, the nature of the association between the Type A personality and serum HDL concentration remains problematic.

In 1996, Denollet's group introduced the Type D personality as a strong coronary risk factor.[10] (Type C relates to coping with cancer.[11,12]) The D stands for a "distressed" personality type—one that has a tendency to experience negative emotions and to inhibit self-expression.[13,14] Patients with coronary artery disease and a Type D personality have a four-fold risk of death compared with non-Type D patients.[15]

Recently, Rozanski and associates extensively reviewed the impact of psychological factors on the pathogenesis of cardiovascular disease.[16] They concluded that psychosocial stressors mediate cardiovascular disease through sympathetic hyperreactivity, enhanced arrhythmogenesis, procoagulant activity, and accelerated atherosclerosis.

How, then, can practitioners use these various findings to help their patients? The answer depends on the medical and psychosocial biases of the individual physician. Friedman and colleagues, for example, helped alter Type A behavior in patients who had sustained a myocardial infarction, contending that such alteration substantially reduces the recurrence of myocardial infarction as well as episodes of silent ischemia.[4,17,18] But is that approach necessarily good? According to a 1981 editorial in *The Lancet*, "making a substantial change in Type A behavior could result in a "demotion in status, in job function, in the regard of colleagues and possibly in personal income."[19]

Despite myriad studies during the past five decades, the precise role of personality types in producing or preventing coronary artery disease awaits clarification. Meanwhile, current evidence suggests that Type D has displaced Type A as the dominant personality risk factor for coronary artery disease. Therefore, to be *B* or not to be *B* is no longer a fitting question. Today, a more appropriate question might be, "Is there any merit in converting the Type A personality to Type B, Type B to A, or Type D to A or B?" All things considered, our answer is an unequivocal... perhaps.

References

[1] Cairns H. The student's objective. Lancet 2:665–66, 1949.

[2] Acierno LJ. Coronary artery disease. *In* The History of Cardiology, Acierno LJ, (Ed). The Parthenon Publishing Group, 1994, p 296.

[3] Friedman M, Rosenman RH. Association of specific overt behavior pattern with blood and cardiovascular findings: Blood

cholesterol level, blood clotting time, incidence of arcus senilis, and clinical coronary artery disease. JAMA 169:1286–96, 1959.

[4] Friedman M, Thoresen CE, Gill JJ, Ulmer D, Thompson L, Powell L, et al. Feasibility of altering type A behavior pattern after myocardial infarction. Recurrent Coronary Prevention Project Study: methods, baseline results, and preliminary findings. Circulation 66:83–92, 1982.

[5] Coronary-prone behavior and coronary heart disease: a critical review. The review panel on coronary-prone behavior and coronary heart disease. Circulation 63:1199–1215, 1981.

[6] Case RB, Heller SS, Case NB, Moss AJ. Type A behavior and survival after acute myocardial infarction. N Engl J Med 312:737–41, 1985.

[7] Kawachi I, Sparrow D, Kubzansky LD, Spiro A, 3rd, Vokonas PS, Weiss ST. Prospective study of a self-report type A scale and risk of coronary heart disease: test of the MMPI-2 type A scale. Circulation 98:405–12, 1998.

[8] Lachar BL. Coronary-prone behavior. Type A behavior revisited. Tex Heart Inst J 20:143–51, 1993.

[9] O'Connor NJ, Manson JE, O'Connor GT, Buring JE. Psychosocial risk factors and nonfatal myocardial infarction. Circulation 92:1458–64, 1995.

[10] Denollet J, Sys SU, Stroobant N, Rombouts H, Gillebert TC, Brutsaert DL. Personality as independent predictor of long-term mortality in patients with coronary heart disease. Lancet 347:417–21, 1996.

[11] Temoshok L, Dreher H. The Type C Connection: The Behavioral Links to Cancer and Your Health. Random House, New York, 1992.

[12] Temoshok L. Complex coping patterns and their role in adaptation and neuroimmunomodulation. Theory, methodology, and research. Ann NY Acad Sci 917: 446–55, 2000.

[13] Denollet J. Type D personality. A potential risk factor refined. J Psychosom Res 49:255–66, 2000.

[14] Denollet J, Van Heck GL. Psychological risk factors in heart disease: what Type D personality is (not) about. J Psychosom Res 51:465–68, 2001.

[15] Denollet J. Personality and coronary heart disease: the type-D scale-16 (DS16). Ann Behav Med 20:209–15, 1998.

[16] Rozanski A, Blumenthal JA, Kaplan J. Impact of psychological factors on the pathogenesis of cardiovascular disease and implications for therapy. Circulation 99:2192–2217, 1999.

[17] Friedman M, Thoresen CE, Gill JJ, Powell LH, Ulmer D, Thompson L et al. Alteration of type A behavior and reduction in cardiac recurrences in postmyocardial infarction patients. Am Heart J 108:237–48, 1984.

[18] Friedman M, Breall WS, Goodwin ML, Sparagon BJ, Ghandour G, Fleischmann N. Effect of type A behavioral counseling on frequency of episodes of silent myocardial ischemia in coronary patients. Am Heart J 132:933–37, 1996.

[19] Are we killing ourselves or not? Lancet 2:669–70, 1981.

The Shakespearean Principle

The scene: Medical teaching rounds in heaven. In attendance are medical students, house officers, and distinguished members of the faculty: Socrates, department chair; Thomas, the Apostle; Publius Vergilius Maro, better known as Virgil; Pyrrho of Elis, founder of Greek Skepticism; and William Shakespeare, department scribe.

SOCRATES: Shall we get started?

HOUSE OFFICER: Today's case is that of an otherwise healthy HIV-positive man who complained of numbness and weakness in his left hand. He denied headache, fever, mental change, visual difficulty, or speech disturbance.

SOCRATES: What did you find on physical examination?

HOUSE OFFICER: Everything was normal except for diminished palmar sensation and weakened grip in the left hand.

SOCRATES: Did you get a CT scan of his head?

HOUSE OFFICER: Yes, that's the first test we did. It showed a 3-cm ring-enhancing lesion with surrounding edema in the right parietal lobe.

SOCRATES: What did the consultants say about that?

HOUSE OFFICER: Neurology, neurosurgery, and neuroradiology all said that toxoplasmosis was the likely diagnosis.

SOCRATES: Why?

VIRGIL: That shouldn't matter. As I've said before, "Always believe the expert."

PYRRHO OF ELIS: Nonsense. As *I've* said before: "Nothing can be known with certainty."

THOMAS, THE APOSTLE: I, too, am inclined to doubt.

SOCRATES: What finally happened?

HOUSE OFFICER: Because I wasn't comfortable with the diagnosis of toxoplasmosis, I began to ask myself some questions.

SOCRATES: *I'll* ask the questions here. What did you ask yourself?

HOUSE OFFICER: I wondered whether the patient could have a neoplasm, a pyogenic abscess, an infarct, or some opportunistic infection. So I did a lumbar puncture.

SOCRATES: And what did you find?

HOUSE OFFICER: There were twenty-one leukocytes, 118 mg/dL of protein, no toxoplasma antibodies, and no cryptococcal antigens. And the fungal, mycobacterial, and routine stains and smears were negative.

SOCRATES: Did you get a spinal fluid VDRL?

HOUSE OFFICER: Yes. It was reactive, 1:4.

SOCRATES: What was the serum RPR?

HOUSE OFFICER: It was 1:1,024. The MHA-TP was also reactive.

SOCRATES: And your conclusion?

HOUSE OFFICER: I decided that the patient probably had a cerebral syphilitic gumma, so I gave him high-dose aqueous penicillin G intravenously for twenty-one days.

SOCRATES: What was the outcome?

HOUSE OFFICER: By day sixteen of therapy, the parietal lobe lesion had almost disappeared. And by day twenty-one, the patient was asymptomatic with a normal physical examination.

SOCRATES: What did you learn from this case?

HOUSE OFFICER: I learned that the right approach to a diagnostic problem can sometimes uncover an answer that had not been considered. And I learned that experts can be wrong.

SOCRATES: Bill, what is our take-home message?

SHAKESPEARE: Let every eye negotiate for itself and trust no agent.

SOCRATES: I can't question that. From now on, let that statement be known as The Shakespearean Principle. And let it be a fundamental doctrine of patient care.

Selected Reading

Berger JR et al. Syphilitic cerebral gumma with HIV infection. Neurology 42:1282, 1992.

Landau WM. Neuroskepticism: Sovereign remedy for the carotid sinus syndrome. Neurology 44:1570, 1994.

Pyrrho of Elis. *In* The Cambridge Encyclopedia, 3rd edn, Crystal D (Ed). Cambridge University Press, New York, 1997, p 878.

Shakespeare W. Much Ado About Nothing. Act II, scene i, line 184.

Virgil. *Æneid* XI.

Wintrobe MM: The virtue of doubt and the spirit of inquiry. Trans Assoc Amer Physicians 78:1, 1965.

Curable Conspicuous Ascites: The Forgotten Four

When conspicuous ascites is the first, the only, or the predominant sign of fluid retention, the doctor should administer thyroid hormone, strip the pericardium, or enter the abdomen!

Absurd as that statement may seem, it highlights the four curable causes of conspicuous ascites that go unrecognized with disconcerting frequency. These "forgotten four" are myxedema; constrictive pericarditis; pancreatitis, usually with pseudocyst formation; and tuberculous peritonitis.

Myxedema

The pathogenesis of ascites in myxedema is unknown. Of the numerous mechanisms postulated, increased capillary permeability seems the most plausible because it could also account for the proteinuria, elevated cerebrospinal fluid protein concentration, and pleural and pericardial effusions that sometimes occur in myxedema. Congestive heart failure might play a role, but in most cases, convincing evidence of cardiac dysfunction is lacking. The ascitic fluid is generally yellow or amber-colored and clear with a protein content ranging from 1.8 to 5.1 gm/dL.

By the time that free intra-abdominal fluid develops, other signs of hypothyroidism are nearly always present. But these signs will be overlooked if the examiner focuses attention only on the abdomen. I have seen nine patients with myxedema ascites, each of whom had a puffy face, low-pitched voice, slow speech, dry skin, and pseudomyotonic deep tendon reflexes. Yet despite such tell-tale physical findings, these patients were misdiagnosed—some for years—as having heart failure, hepatic cirrhosis, or malignancy.

Failure to recognize hypothyroidism as the cause of ascites can be devastating. Some patients have had up to 200 paracenteses before the true nature of their illness became evident. Others have undergone several nondiagnostic exploratory celiotomies. One patient had 460 liters of peritoneal fluid removed over a six-year span. And another had six prolonged hospitalizations and extensive workups for cancer, infection, and liver disease before he died, untreated, from myxedema coma.

Constrictive Pericarditis

Ascites is a prominent early finding in constrictive pericarditis and results from two main factors. Increased systemic venous pressure causes portal hypertension and impedes the return of hepatic lymph. Additionally, the decreased cardiac output reduces renal perfusion, increasing the retention of sodium. Depending on which factor predominates, the ascitic fluid protein concentration will be high (from protein-rich lymph) or low.

Onset of symptoms is typically insidious, and months to years often pass before the correct diagnosis is made. Patients frequently present with decreased muscle mass, hepatomegaly, varying degrees of jaundice, and gross ascites, often with little or no peripheral edema. These findings commonly simulate those of hepatic cirrhosis or abdominal carcinomatosis. Here again, a good physical examination should prevent any diagnostic error. In patients with pericardial constriction, the central venous pressure is elevated and the neck veins are distended. By contrast, in patients with hepatic cirrhosis or abdominal malignancy, the central venous pressure is normal and the neck veins are flat. Making the distinction is crucial, because stripping the pericardium can cure constrictive pericarditis.

Pancreatitis

Patients with pancreatic ascites characteristically have massive amounts of free intra-abdominal fluid, *often without pain.* They also lose appreciable amounts of weight, become markedly weak, and appear chronically ill. The clinical picture, therefore, mimics that of hepatic cirrhosis, tuberculosis, and cancer. To complicate matters, cytologic study of the ascitic fluid in hepatic cirrhosis, tuberculosis, and pancreatitis may give false positive results for malignant cells.

The *sine qua non* for diagnosing pancreatic ascites is a greatly elevated level of ascitic fluid amylase—frequently into the thousands of U/L. Conversely, a normal value exonerates the pancreas as the cause of the ascites. The serum amylase level is usually elevated, but it is always much lower than the amylase level in the ascitic fluid. A normal serum amylase level, however, does not rule out pancreatic ascites.

A leaking pancreatic pseudocyst accounts for the ascites in about two-thirds of these patients. In the remainder, disruption of the pancreatic duct is responsible. Though medical management is sometimes effective, in most patients the condition responds to placement of a stent during endoscopic retrograde cholangio-pancreatography. A few patients require surgical intervention to seal the pancreatic leak.

Tuberculous Peritonitis

Of the curable causes of conspicuous ascites, tuberculous peritonitis is the hardest to establish or exclude. The difficulty stems from a combination of factors: 1) failure to suspect tuberculous peritonitis (perhaps because of its relative rarity and the often normal chest x-ray); 2) the wide spectrum of its clinical manifestations; 3) the variable nature of its ascitic fluid; 4) its frequent association with hepatic cirrhosis; and, most important, 5) failure to obtain peritoneal tissue for histologic examination and culture.

The ascitic fluid may appear clear, greenish-tinged, purulent, or serosanguinous. Rarely, it is chylous or grossly bloody. Acid-fast stains typically are negative, and cultures of the fluid are positive in less than half of the cases. The total and differential leukocyte counts vary widely and can change rapidly. Contrary to popular belief, the fluid may be a transudate, especially in patients with cirrhosis. In fact, the fluid can be physically, chemically, microscopically, and bacteriologically within normal limits.

Measurement of the serum-ascites albumin gradient, the ascitic fluid adenosine deaminase activity, and the ascitic fluid lactic dehydrogenase level has not given consistent findings. And ultrasonography and computed tomography cannot reliably differentiate tuberculous peritonitis from neoplasm or other intra-abdominal inflammatory processes.

Studies from around the world show that laparoscopy or celiotomy is the best way to diagnose tuberculous peritonitis. This approach allows targeted biopsies of the peritoneum, liver, and any abnormal-appearing structure. Even if the peritoneum looks normal or merely thickened, it may still contain granulomas and should be biopsied.

Characteristic laparoscopic appearances include thickened peritoneum with yellow-white miliary tubercles, thickened peritoneum without tubercles, and dense fibrous adhesions gluing various viscera to the peritoneum. These gross findings alone provide sufficient grounds to initiate antituberculous therapy. Biopsy specimens from the peritoneum disclose granulomas, caseating or noncaseating, in 80 percent to 100 percent of the cases. And culture of the biopsy specimens yields the organism in about 75 percent of the cases.

Only Minutes to Hours

These "forgotten four" are curable and thus deserve automatic consideration in every patient with conspicuous ascites, except perhaps those with widespread or terminal malignancy. Moreover, I have observed nine patients who already had histologically proven hepatic cirrhosis in whom long-standing ascites resolved following treatment for coexisting pancreatitis with pseudocyst formation (four), tuberculous peritonitis (two), myxedema (two), and constrictive pericarditis (one).

Three of these four disorders can be effectively ruled in or out within minutes—two by a focused physical examination (myxedema and constrictive pericarditis) and one by measurement of the ascitic fluid amylase content (pancreatitis). And the fourth (tuberculous peritonitis) can be essentially confirmed or excluded within hours—the time it takes for laparoscopy or celiotomy.

In summary, if I have been successful here, my opening statement should no longer seem absurd:

> *When conspicuous ascites is the first, the only, or the predominant sign of fluid retention, the doctor should administer thyroid hormone, strip the pericardium, or enter the abdomen!*

Selected Reading

Bhargava DK et al. Peritoneal tuberculosis: Laparoscopic patterns and its diagnostic accuracy. Am J Gastroenterol 87:109, 1992.

Burack WR, Hollister RM. Tuberculous peritonitis: A study of forty-seven proved cases encountered by a general medical unit in twenty-five years. Am J Med 28:510, 1960.

Cameron JL. Chronic pancreatic ascites and pancreatic pleural effusions. Gastroenterology 74:134, 1978.

Hirschmann JV. Pericardial constriction. Am Heart J 96:110, 1978.

Kocen RS, Atkinson M. Ascites in hypothyroidism. Lancet 1:527, 1963.

Lisehora GE, Margaret Lee Y-T, Barcia PJ. Exploratory laparotomy for diagnosis of tuberculous peritonitis. Surg Gynecol Obstet 169:299, 1989.

Manohar A et al. Symptoms and investigative findings in 145 patients with tuberculous peritonitis diagnosed by peritoneoscopy and biopsy over a five year period. Gut 31:1130, 1990.

Shakil AO et al. Diagnostic features of tuberculous peritonitis in the absence and presence of chronic liver disease: A case control study. Am J Med 100:179, 1996.

Vargas C et al. Diagnostic laparoscopy: A 5-year experience in a hepatology training program. Am J Gastroenterol 90:1258, 1995.

When the Bell Doesn't Ring

Some time ago, a former trainee of mine called long distance to discuss a diagnostic problem.

"I'm stumped," he said. "I've got this forty-three-year-old woman with migratory thrombophlebitis limited to her arms. Initially, I thought she had a painful epitrochlear node, but on resection, the node turned out to be a large thrombosed vein. Similar nodules then appeared on the opposite arm. I've checked her thoroughly for cancer and connective tissue disease, but all tests are negative, and she doesn't respond to anticoagulant or steroid therapy. In fact, lesions developed even while she was receiving steroids."

As I listened, no bell rang. So I asked for more details. In response to my specific questions, he said that the patient was a widow who worked as a nurse's aide in the local hospital. She seemed emotionally stable and gave no history of substance abuse. The lesions were confined almost entirely to the antecubital spaces. They would appear abruptly as small, rounded masses; become red, warm, minimally raised, and tender; grow rapidly to the size of a quarter; and resolve slowly, leaving a sclerotic, ropy base.

In light of this additional information, three things stood out: The doctor was baffled, the lesions were bizarre, and the patient was a female health-care worker with a mystifying ailment. Each of these circumstances alone is enough to suggest factitious disease. Together, they make such diagnosis virtually certain. Other remote considerations would include the nodular form of spontaneous thrombophlebitis, erythema nodosum, subcutaneous fat necrosis, autoerythrocyte sensitization syndrome, Behcet's disease, and a primary infectious process.

Because the initial tissue specimen might not have been adequate or representative of subsequent lesions, I recommended biopsy of a fresh nodule and requested that all slide preparations be sent to me. I then presented them as unknowns to our chief pathologist. He indicated that each showed conspicuously large veins with intensely inflamed, slightly thickened walls surrounding newly formed, non-occluding thrombi. The adjacent fat and overlying skin were normal, and no foreign material or organisms were evident. He wondered whether the patient was a drug addict, and on learning the clinical findings, strongly favored self-induced injury.

When confronted with this new view of her illness, the patient neither admitted nor denied guilt. Nevertheless, her lesions promptly resolved and never recurred.

Diagnostic difficulty in this case arose because the doctor did what all of us do from time to time—he focused on a part and lost sight of the whole. By zeroing in on thrombophlebitis, he couldn't see the link between his own puzzlement, the strikingly finite location of the lesions, and the patient's gender and health-related occupation—a combination classic for factitious disease.

Moral: When the right diagnostic bell doesn't ring, you may be in the wrong belfry.

Selected Reading

Aduan RP et al. Factitious fever and self-induced infection: A report of 32 cases and review of the literature. Ann Intern Med 90:230, 1979.

Montgomery H, O'Leary PA, Barker NW. Nodular vascular diseases of the legs: Erythema induratum and allied conditions. JAMA 128:335, 1945.

Reich P, Gottfried LA. Factitious disorders in a teaching hospital. Ann Intern Med 99:240, 1983.

Weinstein L. Erythema nodosum. Dis Mon, June:1, 1984.

Five Cases in Search of a Diagnostician

An ever-spreading malady is undermining our profession. I call it *technologic tenesmus*—the uncontrollable urge to rely on sophisticated medical gadgetry for diagnosis. It typically strikes the ill-trained and ill-informed but endangers all of us. Particularly susceptible are those who lack self-confidence, fear litigation, or are looking for ways to bypass the medical history, physical examination, and time required for thinking.

As a result of this malady, health care costs are soaring, the fun and challenge of medicine are disappearing, and the doctor-patient relationship is becoming depersonalized. And unless we find a cure, tomorrow's physicians will never gain proficiency in using the best tool they have—the brain.

Protection against technologic tenesmus requires frequent use of one's mind. To that end, I present five puzzling cases. Four of the patients I knew as a senior student or intern in 1954; the other I cared for in 1968. I missed the diagnosis in every case. Let's see how you do.

Case Presentations

CASE 1. A fifty-seven-year-old man was admitted to the hospital because of fever, chills, chest pain, and a right pleural effusion. Aside from frequent alcoholic binges, he had been well until two months earlier, when he experienced constant dull epigastric pain for a week. Chest x-ray and extensive workup of his gastrointestinal tract demonstrated no abnormality.

Six weeks before admission, he had had shaking chills and fever that disappeared after his private physician treated him with a broad-spectrum antibiotic. Two weeks before admission, he noticed dull, right-sided anterolateral chest pain that soon became pleuritic and radiated to his right shoulder. Fever and chills recurred, this time accompanied by a nonproductive cough. These symptoms persisted, prompting him to seek medical help.

On physical examination, the man appeared chronically ill. He had dullness to percussion and diminished breath sounds over the lower part of his right lung. No other abnormalities were evident.

Routine studies of his blood, urine, and liver function were normal. Right thoracentesis yielded clear pleural fluid with a protein content of 4.7 gm/dL, many lymphocytes and histiocytes, but no malignant cells. Bronchoscopy showed purulent secretions arising from the right lower lobe bronchus. Cultures of blood, pleural fluid, and bronchial washings were negative. Needle biopsy of the pleura showed chronic inflammation. Oral cholecystography and barium x-ray examination of the entire gastrointestinal tract demonstrated no abnormality. Hepatic scanning using gold 198 showed an area of diminished isotope concentration in the posterior aspect of the dome of the liver.

CASE 2. A twenty-five-year-old previously healthy woman was brought to the hospital by her husband after she had had a generalized tonic-clonic seizure. On arrival, she was alert and oriented but complained of paresthesias of her face, fingers, and toes. The only abnormal physical finding was bilateral papilledema. X-rays of her chest and skull were normal. Lumbar puncture yielded clear spinal fluid under normal pressure, with normal amounts of protein and sugar and no cells.

CASE 3. A robust forty-year-old butcher and bird fancier camped out overnight. The next morning he removed a tick from his abdomen. For breakfast he ate poorly cooked pork sausage and drank water from a stream adjacent to an outhouse. Then, while trekking through the woods, he stepped on a rusty nail, puncturing the skin of his foot. Next he killed and skinned a wild rabbit. Early that afternoon, he felt febrile, noticed generalized myalgia and arthralgia, and decided to go to the hospital. On arrival, he appeared acutely ill. His temperature was 39.4 C, and he had a few red spots on his chest. He rapidly became disoriented and within hours lapsed into a coma.

CASE 4. A sixty-five-year-old man complained of difficulty starting his urinary stream. On physical examination, he appeared to be healthy, and the only abnormal finding was an enlarged prostate. Results of routine laboratory studies were normal. An intravenous urogram, however, showed minimal bilateral hydronephrosis. The patient then had a transurethral prostatectomy under spinal anesthesia. The operation went smoothly, recovery was rapid, and the resected tissue was benign, but his urinary problem persisted. Review of the case uncovered a peculiar fact: In the operative record, the anesthesiologist had described the patient's spinal fluid as being dark yellow.

CASE 5. A thirty-five-year-old woman was admitted to the hospital because of cough and chest pain of four months' duration. She said she had been well until ten months earlier, when she took quinine to induce an abortion. Soon thereafter, she had been admitted to a hospital because of uterine bleeding, abdominal cramps, and fever. Her symptoms resolved after forceps removal of a piece of partially expelled placenta, but two weeks later, fever and abdominal cramps recurred, prompting another hospitalization. At that time she had a tender right adnexal mass, a purulent cervical discharge, and a small, freely movable uterus. After ten days of antibiotic therapy, she felt well and had normal menstrual periods.

Four months before the second admission, she had abrupt onset of a nonproductive cough associated with left-sided chest pain.

These symptoms waxed and waned, and a few weeks later, a chest x-ray showed an infiltrate in the lower part of the left lung. Three months before admission, her cough became persistent, her chest pain became pleuritic, and the tips of her fingers and toes gradually enlarged. Then one month before admission, she began to cough up large amounts of foul-tasting yellow sputum accompanied by shortness of breath, night sweats, and fatigue.

At admission, she appeared chronically ill. She had fever, rales at the base of the left lung, and clubbing of her fingers and toes. The findings on pelvic examination were normal. Laboratory studies showed a normochromic, normocytic anemia. Total leukocyte count, urinalysis, and bone marrow examination were normal. Sputum was mucopurulent, with no predominant organisms. Chest x-ray showed an indistinct density in the left lower lung field near the cardiac apex. Bronchography and bronchoscopy were noncontributory. Despite a month of postural drainage, steam inhalation, and therapy with oxytetracycline and penicillin, her condition failed to improve.

Diagnoses

CASE 1: TOOTHPICK PLEURISY. Exploratory thoracotomy disclosed a toothpick embedded in the posterolateral portion of the diaphragm and extending into the lower lobe of the adjacent lung. Dense adhesions and a small pocket of pus surrounded the toothpick. After removal of the foreign body and decortication of the affected pulmonary tissue, the patient recovered rapidly. When repeatedly questioned after the operation, he could not recall having swallowed the toothpick.

Lesson: Toothpicks as foreign bodies are especially dangerous because they are sharp at both ends, indigestible, and radiographically undetectable. Once ingested, they may pass through the bowel wall, causing peritonitis or abscess formation at or distal to the site of perforation.

This patient presumably swallowed the toothpick during an alcoholic binge. It then perforated the bowel, migrated to the subdiaphragmatic space, worked its way partially through the diaphragm into the lung, and caused perhaps the first case of pleural disease attributable to ingestion of a toothpick.

CASE 2: IDIOPATHIC HYPOPARATHYROIDISM. This case baffled everyone except Frank Tyler, then Chief of Endocrinology and Metabolism at the University of Utah School of Medicine. After hearing the story and examining the patient, he suspected hypoparathyroidism and ordered measurement of serum calcium and phosphorus. The results confirmed his suspicions—hypocalcemia and hyperphosphatemia. With calcium supplementation and vitamin D therapy, the papilledema resolved and seizures did not occur.

Lesson: Seizures or papilledema or both may signal idiopathic or postoperative hypoparathyroidism. Failure to appreciate this can lead to fruitless and potentially dangerous investigations, depriving the patient of specific, corrective treatment. The cause of the papilledema is uncertain, but with appropriate replacement therapy, the papilledema resolves. Lumbar puncture in these patients commonly yields fluid under increased pressure, suggesting pseudotumor cerebri. But, as in the case presented, the spinal fluid pressure may be normal. It is prudent, therefore, to obtain a serum calcium level in any patient with unexplained seizures or papilledema, particularly when carpopedal spasm or paresthesias also are present.

CASE 3: MENINGOCOCCAL MENINGITIS AND BACTEREMIA. Because of the incredible exposure history, the house officers and students familiar with this patient offered a variety of diagnoses: brucellosis, psittacosis, trichinosis, typhoid fever, tetanus, tularemia, and Rocky Mountain spotted fever (Lyme disease was unknown at that time). I favored typhoid fever with rose spots.

Shortly after the patient's admission, the intern who initially examined him presented the case to Ivan L. Bennett, Jr., a visiting professor from Yale University School of Medicine. After examining the patient, Bennett made this unforgettable statement: "Excluding drugs and trauma, only two things can put a perfectly healthy person into a coma in less than twenty-four hours. One is spontaneous intracranial hemorrhage; the other is meningococcal infection." He then asked the intern to do a gram stain of an aspirate from one of the red spots on the patient's chest. It showed gram-negative intracellular diplococci. Cultures of blood, cerebrospinal fluid, and aspirate all grew *Neisseria meningitidis.* The patient died despite penicillin therapy.

Lesson: With rare exceptions, Bennett's dictum still holds true. Indeed, meningococcemia, with or without meningitis, can be fulminating, with death occurring in less than two hours after the first symptom appears. Petechiae, especially on the extremities, are characteristic of this infection. This case also illustrates the importance of considering the incubation period when diagnosing specific infectious diseases. In that regard, none of the diagnoses put forth by the students and house officers fitted the overall clinical picture.

CASE 4: SPINAL CORD TUMOR. Confused by the finding of dark yellow spinal fluid, I consulted Len Jarcho, Chief of Neurology at the University of Utah School of Medicine. He elicited from the patient a history of recent low back pain and difficulty defecating. On physical examination, Jarcho found hypoesthesia in the saddle region along with diminished anal and bulbocavernosus reflexes. He then diagnosed Froin syndrome—xanthochromic spinal fluid consequent to cord compression by tumor. A subsequent myelogram showed an intradural extramedullary mass with block in the lumbar area. The patient had a benign tumor removed from his cauda equina, after which he regained normal function of his bladder and rectum.

Lesson: Xanthochromic spinal fluid has three basic causes: hemorrhage into the spinal canal, hyperbilirubinemia (serum total bilirubin level usually above 10 mg/dL), and cord compression blocking the flow of spinal fluid. The patient's clinical manifestations and serum bilirubin level should point immediately to the probable mechanism and to the type and extent of further workup.

With hemorrhage into the spinal canal, the yellow color results from hemoglobin or its breakdown products; with jaundice, the pigment is bilirubin. In patients with cord compression, the pigment also is bilirubin, but the spinal fluid protein concentration is strikingly elevated as well (generally greater than 1,000 mg/dL).

Besides showing how important yellow spinal fluid is, this case teaches another lesson: Things are not always what they seem. Initially, the patient's obstructive uropathy appeared to be an obvious consequence of prostatic hypertrophy. His prostatic hypertrophy, however, was purely coincidental. Had I taken a better history and done a better physical examination, I might have suspected a neurologic cause for the patient's problem.

CASE 5: FOREIGN BODY IN THE LUNG. To the amazement of everyone connected with this case, exploratory thoracotomy unveiled a foot-long woven silk catheter embedded in the lingula and extending for some distance into the left upper lobe. The catheter also extended over the pleura of the left lower lobe and through the diaphragm into the abdominal cavity. After the operation, the patient admitted that another person had aborted her pregnancy, using a catheter, but she thought that the catheter had been removed.

Lesson: Anything can happen in medicine. Who would have thought that a catheter could enter the vagina, leave the uterus, and then in a span of about five months wend its way through the abdominal cavity, pierce the diaphragm, and lodge in the lung? Aside from case 1, I could find only one other example of a foreign body (a 40 x 30 cm surgical sponge) that somehow migrated into the lung from below the diaphragm. The present case also reminds us that patients sometimes lie. But even if this patient had told the truth about her abortion, I doubt that anyone could have predicted the findings at thoracotomy.

Final Comments

In cases 1 and 5, nothing short of surgical exploration could have established the exact cause of illness. By contrast, in cases 2, 3, and 4, veteran clinicians made the correct diagnosis at the bedside. They did not require computed tomography, magnetic resonance imaging, ultrasonography, or any other sophisticated diagnostic technology to initiate or substantiate their impressions. They relied on the best diagnostic tool they had—the brain.

Selected Reading

Snodgrass TJ. Foreign bodies in the intestinal tract. Arch Surg 55:441, 1947.

Jenson AB, Fred HL. Toothpick pleurisy (letter). JAMA 203:988, 1968.

Bajandas FJ, Smith JL. Optic neuritis in hypoparathyroidism. Neurology 26:451, 1976.

Dimich A, Bedrossian PB, Wallach S. Hypoparathyroidism: Clinical observations in 34 patients. Arch Intern Med 120:449, 1967.

Sheldon RS et al. Hypoparathyroidism and pseudotumor cerebri: An infrequent clinical association. Can J Neurol Sci 14:622, 1987.

Magnussen CR. Work-up for sudden fever and shock in a previously healthy adult: Key clues to differentiating six deadly, fulminant infections. J Crit Illness 6:421, 1991.

Cole JT, Flaum MA. Postsplenectomy infections. South Med J 85:1220, 1992.

Giraud T et al. Adult overwhelming meningococcal purpura: A study of 35 cases, 1977–1989. Arch Intern Med 151:310, 1991.

Feldman HA. Recent developments in the therapy and control of meningococcal infections. Dis Mon 2:1, 1966.

Rosenberg DG, Galambos JT. Yellow spinal fluid: Diagnostic significance of cerebrospinal fluid in jaundiced patients. Am J Dig Dis 5:32, 1960.

Barrows LJ, Hunter FT, Banker BQ. The nature and clinical significance of pigments in the cerebrospinal fluid. Brain 78:59, 1955.

Xanthochromia (editorial). Lancet 2:658, 1989.

Barnes AC, Boitnott JK: Clinicopathologic conference. Johns Hopkins Med J 120:420, 1967.

Molinari P, Acrich M, Casco MR. Migration of a foreign body into the lung: Case report. Dis Chest 45:428, 1964.

LOOKING BACK

...feeling a big gallbladder at the bedside should be more gratifying than finding it first by ultrasonography, computerized tomographic scanning, or magnetic resonance imaging. Which brings me to this question: Would you know a gallbladder if you felt one?

–H. L. F. in "Courvoisier Revisited"

So, if we keep our eyes open, our minds in gear, and our thoracentesis trays handy, Contarini's condition could rise from obscurity to become a household name.

–H. L. F. in "Contarini's Condition"

Looking Back

Medicine has changed—from a highly respected calling to a big-time business. In the process, the practice of medicine has also changed. We physicians previously used our minds and five senses to make diagnoses. Today we use machines. Formerly, we put our thoughts in order before we ordered tests; now we order tests to generate our thoughts. A good medical history and a careful physical examination used to be routine. But these days, we routinely get a blood gas in place of examining the lungs, obtain an echocardiogram instead of listening to the heart, and rely on consultants rather than ourselves for important medical decisions.

Because of these many changes, the coveted patient-doctor bond has weakened, the lawyer-patient relationship has strengthened, and medicine has lost its fun—at least for me. As a consequence, I find myself often looking back—back to the time when medicine *was* fun.

In those days, we focused on the patient, not the laboratory. We understood the pathophysiology, clinical features, and natural history of diseases. We took pride in developing and maintaining our bedside skills. And we welcomed diagnostic challenges.

Join me as I revisit a few of my patients from that era. Given their case histories, what would your diagnoses be?

Case Presentations

CASE 1. A Ute Indian underwent drainage of a perirectal abscess. During the next few months, he experienced asymptomatic, odorless destruction of his entire perineum and scrotum. The process eventually laid bare his testes and ischial bones. Repeated biopsies and cultures of the affected tissues shed no light on the cause, and despite administration of multiple antibiotics, he died.

CASE 2. A generalized purple hue and lanugo-type facial hair developed in a middle-aged white woman. Within nine months, her entire skin had turned black.

CASE 3. An elderly woman had a knee that was distinctly warm to the touch but normal in appearance and painless. These findings did not change during three years of follow-up.

CASE 4. A healthy young woman complained of increasing difficulty reading fine print. While testing her strength, I had her squeeze my hand. It took her five seconds to let go.

CASE 5. Two vagrants hopped a freight train in Reno, Nevada—drunk, but otherwise O.K. On arriving in Salt Lake City the next day, one was dead and the other was blind.

CASE 6. A young man had shortness of breath and what appeared to be a pulsating testicle.

CASE 7. A boy could smile but he could not whistle.

Diagnoses

CASE 1: CUTANEOUS AMEBIASIS. Autopsy of this patient uncovered no explanation for his death. Several months later, however, the *Annals of Internal Medicine* published a picture of a man whose ulcerated perineum looked just like the perineum of my patient. The diagnosis in that case was cutaneous amebiasis. I immediately contacted the staff pathologist who had interpreted the premortem biopsy specimens and autopsy material from my patient. Through the retrospectoscope—our best teaching instrument—he found amebic trophozoites in virtually all of the histologic sections.

Cutaneous amebiasis deserves consideration in any patient with extensive necrosis and ulceration of the skin and underlying tissues. Amebic trophozoites are easy to miss in sections stained by hematoxylin and eosin; they also are easily confused with macrophages.

CASE 2. MALIGNANT MELANOMA. At autopsy this woman had widespread metastases with intense deposits of melanin throughout her skin and internal organs. Malignant melanoma is the only condition known to turn a white person's entire skin absolutely black. This patient's lanugo-type facial hair was an early cutaneous marker of internal malignancy.

CASE 3. PAGET'S DISEASE OF BONE. An x-ray of the knee showed cortical thickening, coarsened trabeculae, and areas of lucency in the distal femur. Paget's disease is associated with increased regional blood flow up to twenty times greater than normal; this may result in warm limbs and reddish skin in the involved areas. Pain is often absent, and affected joints need not be enlarged or deformed.

CASE 4. MYOTONIC DYSTROPHY. The cardinal feature of this disease is persistence of muscle contraction after active motion. Typically, patients cannot quickly open the hand after making a fist. In addition, they frequently have a distinctive type of cataract that affects their vision.

CASE 5. METHYL ALCOHOL POISONING. The survivor admitted that he and his buddy had drunk illicit whiskey the previous day, but he couldn't remember what happened after that. On examination, he was acidotic, with hyperemic optic discs and retinal edema—findings classic for methyl alcohol intoxication.

CASE 6. TRICUSPID INSUFFICIENCY WITH VARICOCELE. Testicles don't pulsate, but varicoceles can. Pulsatile varicose veins anywhere in the body are pathognomonic of tricuspid insufficiency. The patient in question had rheumatic heart disease. (Another patient of mine had a pulsating varicocele associated with the tricuspid insufficiency of Ebstein's anomaly.)

CASE 7. FACIOSCAPULOHUMERAL MUSCULAR DYSTROPHY. Diffuse involvement of the facial muscles is a striking feature of this disorder. Asymmetric involvement of the orbicularis oris results in an inability to pucker the lips, thereby prohibiting whistling.

If you considered the right diagnosis in all of these cases, you deserve a medal. But even if you missed a few—as I did back then—I hope you had fun.

Selected Reading

Bennett IL Jr et al. Acute methyl alcohol poisoning: A review based on experiences in an outbreak of 323 cases. Medicine 32:431, 1953.

Brickner PW, Scudder WT, Weinrib M. Pulsating varicose veins in functional tricuspid insufficiency: Case report and venous pressure tracing. Circulation 25:126, 1962.

Burian HM, Burns CA. Ocular changes in myotonic dystrophy. Am J Ophthalmol 63:22, 1967.

Davson J, Jones DM, Turner L. Diagnosis of Meleney's synergistic gangrene. Br J Surg 75:267, 1988.

Fitzpatrick TB, Montgomery H, Lerner AB. Pathogenesis of generalized dermal pigmentation secondary to malignant melanoma and melanuria. J Invest Dermatol 22:163, 1954.

Franck WA et al. Rheumatic manifestations of Paget's disease of bone. Am J Med 56:592, 1974.

McConaghey RMS. Amoebiasis of the anus and perineum: With report of a case. Indian Medical Gazette 80:79, 1945.
Perkoff GT, Tyler FH. The differential diagnosis of progressive muscular dystrophy. Med Clin North Am 37:545, 1953.
Rhodes BA et al. Absence of anatomic arteriovenous shunts in Paget's disease of bone. New Engl J Med 287:686, 1972.
Song YS. Cutaneous amebiasis: Report of two cases with one autopsy. Ann Intern Med 44:1211, 1956.
Trueblood DV. Malignant melanoma with generalized skin blackening: The white girl who turned black. Northwest Med 46:199, 1947.
Wadskov S. Bro-Jørgensen A, Søndergaard J. Acquired hypertrichosis lanuginosa: A skin marker of internal malignancy. Arch Dermatol 112:1442, 1976.

Courvoisier Revisited

> "For this study, I have divided 187 cases into 2 main groups: 87 obstructions due to stone and 100 due to other causes. In those due to stone, 80.4 percent revealed a shrunken gallbladder and 19.6 percent revealed a dilated gallbladder. In obstruction due to other causes, the gallbladder is seldom shrunken (8 out of 100 cases), the majority (92 out of 100 cases) being dilated. In other words, *with stone obstruction of the common duct dilatation of the gallbladder is rare. Usually the organ is already shrunken. With obstruction due to other causes, dilatation is most common, atrophy occurring in only one-twelfth of the cases.*"
>
> "Consequently we have an important diagnostic point in the differential diagnosis of common duct obstruction."[1]

That study, done at autopsy more than a century ago, earned Ludwig Georg Courvoisier a niche in medical history. Unfortunately, his conclusions are frequently misquoted and his findings misinterpreted or misapplied. Complicating matters are numerous eponyms, each with a different meaning and each with a different connotation—Courvoisier's "law,"[2-5] "sign,"[2,6-8] "gallbladder,"[6,9] "hypothesis," [6,9] "phenomenon,"[2] and "syndrome."[6] No wonder controversy and confusion shroud this pioneering work. But first, a note about the pioneer.

Courvoisier was born in Basel, Switzerland, in 1843.[2,5] Contrary to popular belief, he wasn't French, as his last name suggests. He was a German national who actually fought against France during the Franco-Prussian War.[2,5,8] As a child, he acquired an interest in botany and entomology and later became a recognized expert in those sciences.[5,8] He went to medical school in Basel, where he had a private practice, served as Professor of Surgery in the local university, and died of pneumonia in 1918.[2,5,8]

The conclusions that Courvoisier drew from his study pertain strictly to patients with common duct obstruction.[1] Failure to appreciate this point has contributed to the confusion surrounding his work. For example, his findings don't apply when the common duct is normal, even if jaundice and an enlarged gallbladder are present.[10] And they don't apply when cholecystomegaly exists in the absence of jaundice and common duct obstruction.[7]

Some writers argue that although Courvoisier was as accurate as he could be in his time, "The Law is now of little use...."[3] Indeed, recent evidence indicates that distensibility of the gallbladder correlates more closely with the degree and duration of elevated intraductal pressure than with inflammation and scarring as Courvoisier proposed.[9] Additionally, some investigators contend that a palpable gallbladder is of little value in differentiating benign from malignant causes of obstructive jaundice.[4] Others believe that the predictive value of a palpable gallbladder in jaundiced patients depends on the incidence of gallstones and cancer in the population being treated.[5]

Controversy and confusion aside, Courvoisier did much to advance our knowledge of biliary tract disease. And thanks to him, clinicians have reason to become adept at detecting an enlarged gallbladder by physical examination. After all, feeling a big gallbladder at the bedside should be more gratifying than finding it first by ultrasonography, computerized tomographic scanning, or magnetic resonance imaging. Which brings me to this question: Would you know a gallbladder if you felt one?

References

[1] Courvoisier LG. *Kasuistisch-Statistische Beiträge zur Pathologie und Chirurgie der Gallenwege.* Vogel, Leipzig, 1890, pp 57–58.

[2] Morgenstern L, Ludwig G. Courvoisier and Courvoisier's law. Surg Gynecol Obstet 110:383–84, 1960.

[3] Watts GT. Courvoisier's law. Lancet 2:1293–94, 1985.

[4] Viteri AL. Courvoisier's law and evaluation of the jaundiced patient. Tex Med 76:60–61, 1985.

[5] Verghese A, Dison C, Berk SL. Courvoisier's "law"—An eponym in evolution. Am J Gastroenterol 82:248–50, 1987.

[6] Delpre G, Kadish U. Courvoisier's gallbladder: "Render unto Caesar that which is Caesar's." Dig Dis Sci 32:446, 1987.

[7] Fournier AM, Michel J. Courvoisier's sign revisited: Two patients with palpable gallbladder. South Med J 85:548–50, 1992.

[8] Anonymous. Ludwig Courvoisier (1843–1918): Courvoisier's sign. JAMA 204:165, 1968.

[9] Chung RS. Pathogenesis of the "Courvoisier gallbladder." Dig Dis Sci 28:33–38, 1983.

[10] Eiband JM, Fred HL, Jordan GL Jr. Jaundice and enlargement of the gallbladder: A diagnostic problem. Report of 2 cases. Am J Dig Dis 11:664–68, 1966.

Contarini's Condition

Attention aficionados of medical arcana. Here's one whose clinical relevance could be greater today than ever before. It is *Contarini's condition.*

Francesco Contarini (1556–1624) was the ninety-fifth Doge of the Venetian Republic. Details of his fatal illness and autopsy appeared in a case report by Velschius in 1667; centuries later, Jarcho[1] resurrected that report and quoted extensively from it.

> [H]e developed a fever which had the character of a double tertian and returned, sometimes ahead of schedule for a few days and sometimes delayed for an equal length of time or even longer.... The patient also had a mild little cough, by which he brought up a small amount of thick phlegm. His breathing was quite free. However it was hard for him to lie on either side.

After several months of intermittent fever and slight cough, the Doge experienced sudden difficulty breathing. "He had to sleep almost upright and could not rest on either side.... With difficulty he spat up thick ashen and yellowish matter that resembled something rotten." A few days later, Contarini died. At autopsy,

> the cavity of the chest contained about five pounds of watery matter. The flaccid right part of the lung appeared to be full of thick mucous fluid. The left had turned entirely into a whitish gore, which was contained in the

> pulmonary tunic as if in a sac. When this was cut apart, about 16 ounces of matter flowed out into the thoracic cavity. No trace of lung remained on the left side except the mark of the membrane which adhered to the ribs. The heart was very large but was not contaminated by matter either internally or externally.

From these findings Jarcho concluded that Contarini had suffered right-sided hydrothorax consequent to congestive heart failure and left-sided lung abscess or empyema.

In 1978, Kutty and Varkey[2] presented the case of a man with leukemia who had a right-sided sterile pleural effusion. They attributed the effusion to his leukemia and concomitant cardiac failure. Two weeks later, follow-up chest roentgenogram showed bilateral pleural effusions, more notable on the left. Persistent low-grade fever prompted left-sided thoracentesis which "yielded a pure heavy growth of coagulase-positive *[Staphylococcus] aureus.*" Spurred by Jarcho's account, Kutty and Varkey coined *Contarini's condition,* defining it as bilateral pleural effusions with markedly different characteristics. They suggested that patients who have bilateral pleural effusions and are receiving immunotherapy are prime candidates for bilateral diagnostic thoracenteses, particularly if unexplained fever coexists.

I have recognized *Contarini's condition* primarily in patients with cardiac failure who had a serous transudate on one side and pulmonary infarction causing a bloody exudate on the opposite side. A striking exception, however, was that of an elderly man with well-differentiated lymphocytic malignant lymphoma. His chest roentgenogram demonstrated a large, left pleural effusion. At thoracentesis, the effusion was grossly bloody, sterile, and laden with lymphocytes histologically consistent with lymphocytic lymphoma. Two months later, another chest roentgenogram showed large pleural effusions bilaterally. The fluid on the left was unchanged in color and composition; on the right, it was chylous and

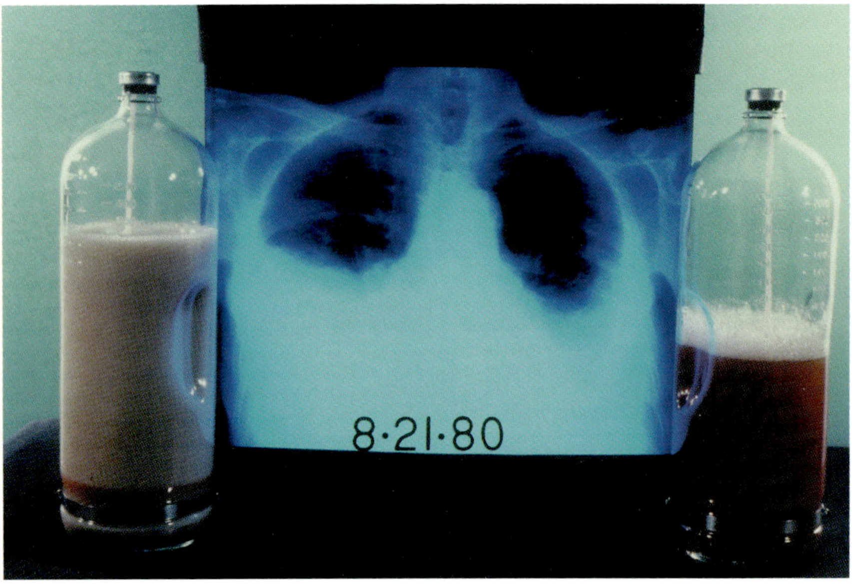
8·21·80

almost devoid of cells (See Figure). In this case, the asynchronous development of the effusions offered a clue to their disparate nature.

A search of the English-language medical literature from 1979 through 1990 uncovered no reference to *Contarini's condition.* This situation may change, however, considering the propensity of patients with AIDS to manifest, in combination, diverse intrathoracic complications. So, if we keep our eyes open, our minds in gear, and our thoracentesis trays handy, *Contarini's condition* could rise from obscurity to become a household name.

Seek, and ye shall find.
–Matthew 7:7

References

[1] Jarcho S. Empyema or hydrothorax in the ninety-fifth doge of Venice. Bull NY Acad Med 46:378–85, 1970.

[2] Kutty CPK, Varkey B. "Contarini's condition": bilateral pleural effusions with markedly different characteristics. Chest 74:679–80, 1978.

The Clinicopathological Conference

The clinicopathological conference, known throughout the English-speaking medical world as the CPC, is a time-honored and widely accepted means of teaching and learning differential diagnosis. I wonder, however, whether many physicians today are familiar with its history, ever think about its drawbacks, or can recognize the changes it has undergone over the years. In this editorial, I address these matters and comment on the benefits and future of the CPC.

History of the Conference

> *The idea of using printed records of cases as centres of interest in studying medicine occurred to me some two years ago. Since that time I have been watching carefully for every possible opportunity to apply the method, and have tried to see all the objections which might be raised against the plan. It was only when I was fully convinced that a study of real histories could be made feasible in teaching medicine that the scheme was brought forward.*

Those are the words of Walter B. Cannon, a medical student at Harvard, and later a professor of physiology there. He was speaking before the Boston Society for Medical Improvement on 5 March 1900. The general subject of discussion that day was "Some Advances in Medical Education." Cannon had gotten the idea of case-based teaching from his roommate, a student at Harvard Law School. In a report published two months earlier, Cannon had said that law students "...learn their law not by dreary grubbing at textbooks or lecture notes, but by vigorously 'threshing out a case' with one another" (as in a mock trial).

Later that same year, Richard C. Cabot, a prominent Harvard internist, put Cannon's proposal into action by initiating case-oriented teaching exercises in his private office. Ultimately, these conferences moved to the Massachusetts General Hospital, where they were known as the Cabot Case Records. In 1924, *The Boston Medical and Surgical Journal* started publishing the conferences. Four years later, that journal became *The New England Journal of Medicine,* in which CPCs have been a feature ever since.

Soon after its birth in Boston, the CPC took root in other cities across the country. In Baltimore, at the Johns Hopkins Medical School, CPCs were conducted for many years by a famous duo: William Thayer (clinician) and William McCallum (pathologist). By 1950, when I arrived there as a student, the chairman of medicine, A. McGehee Harvey, and the chairman of pathology, Arnold Rich, had assumed command of the conferences. Every Wednesday at noon, a host of students, house officers, and faculty members crammed into a dimly lit, smoke-filled room to hear these two giants match wits. The opportunity to observe their analytical minds in action on a regular basis for four straight years was an unforgettable privilege for me.

One other historical figure deserves mention. William Dock was a brilliant educator and master clinician who had a decisive influence on American medicine for more than half of this century. In his heyday, he would travel to various medical centers to serve as visiting professor. Part of his role on such occasions was to be the discussant at the CPC. But in sharp contrast to virtually all other discussants, he preferred not to see the protocol until he had entered the conference room and was ready to begin. Then, standing before a sophisticated audience of highly educated physicians, he would read the protocol aloud, pausing after each sentence to verbalize his analysis of the information it contained. Immediately after reading the last line, he would announce his final diagnosis. Amazingly, he usually nailed it. (I tried his approach once and failed miserably.)

Benefits

Deductive reasoning and clinicopathological correlation are linchpins of the CPC, and no other educational exercise so effectively combines factual information with an organized, step-by-step approach to clinical problem solving. The primary purpose is *not* to showcase a virtuoso diagnostic performance but to illustrate a logical, instructive analysis of the available evidence. It doesn't matter so much in CPCs if the diagnosis is wrong as long as the *approach* to the diagnosis is right. In other words, getting the wrong diagnosis for the right reasons is better than getting the right diagnosis for the wrong reasons. Failure to understand or accept this principle greatly reduces the benefits of the CPC.

Besides being the paradigm for clinical problem solving, the CPC offers other, less obvious benefits. It helps students realize that their professors are not always right. It helps young discussants appreciate the difficulty of analyzing clinical information correctly. It helps all discussants become better teachers. And it helps doctors overcome the fear of being wrong.

Drawbacks

Under the rules of the CPC, discussants cannot question or examine the patient. Nor can they order tests and procedures of their choice. Consequently, they must work with the information given them—information filtered through the eyes and brains of others. But if that information is inadequate or inaccurate, or when it is altered intentionally to make the case more challenging, the discussant's analysis will be based on false premises and will be likely to lead to erroneous conclusions.

Discussants at CPCs typically spend many hours—sometimes days or even weeks—studying the protocol, reading pertinent literature, formulating a differential diagnosis, and preparing their remarks. That approach to clinical problem solving is fine for CPCs, but few practicing physicians can afford such luxury.

Many times, discussants go overboard by considering at length every conceivable diagnostic possibility. At other times, they correctly limit the differential diagnosis but get bogged down in minutiae. These seemingly erudite approaches obscure the essence of the case and diminish its teaching value.

Improper case selection is another way that CPCs get an undeserved black eye. The most damaging impropriety is selecting a case chiefly to tease or embarrass the discussant. Another is selecting a case in which no one could make the correct diagnosis from the evidence presented. In both instances, the case usually represents a condition that is rare, bizarre, or newly described; in other words, it does not reflect an everyday clinical problem. And such cases keep alive the lingering belief that CPCs are guessing games involving trickery.

Changes

Advances in diagnostic technology have shifted the focus of medicine from the bedside to the laboratory. As a consequence, today's CPCs differ in many not-so-obvious ways from those in the first half or more of this century.

To begin with, the case material is somewhat different. Answers formerly available only at autopsy are now often evident from imaging studies, endoscopic examinations, or fine needle biopsies. Thus, diseases such as liver abscess, pancreatic carcinoma, and subdural hematoma—frequent culprits in CPCs of yesteryear—rarely qualify for CPCs today. Moreover, in years past, the CPC protocol primarily emphasized the patient's medical history, physical examination, and hospital course. Nowadays, laboratory data take center stage.

The main participants in CPCs have also changed. For many years, the same clinician and pathologist usually conducted the conferences, no matter what disease the patient had. These days, the clinician and pathologist vary according to the subspecialty into which the case fits.

Finally, the frequency and popularity of CPCs are waning. Early on, CPCs were unquestionably the weekly highlight of educational activities in most, if not all, of our medical schools. Although they still take place in many medical centers, they do not necessarily occur weekly or regularly, and they are not always well attended. Thankfully, they do still appear in print—almost every week in *The New England Journal of Medicine,* every other month in the *American Journal of Medicine,* and occasionally in *Circulation.*

The Future

Someone once said, "Judging from the way things look, it's a good thing the future doesn't come all at once." Well, the way things look in medicine these days, the future of the CPC seems bleak—at least to me. And if Cannon and Cabot were still alive, they would probably agree. The glory days of the CPC appear to be over—master clinicians are almost extinct, bedside skills are neither fashionable nor commonly sought, treatment has overtaken diagnosis as a priority in medical education, and the medical profession has become more of a business than a calling.

On the positive side, our understanding of disease and our ability to care for the sick are better than ever. So the need for CPCs may not be as great as it once was. Nevertheless, until doctors are no longer necessary for health care, I believe that a well-planned CPC will continue to be a worthwhile educational activity. After all, where else can we exercise an important part of our body without buying expensive equipment, risking serious injury, or upsetting our spouse?

Selected Reading

Cannon WB. The case method of teaching systematic medicine. Boston Med & Surg J 142:31, 1900.

Cannon WB. The case system in medicine. Boston Med & Surg J 142:563, 1900.

Castleman B, Dudley HR Jr. Clinicopathological Conferences of the Massachusetts General Hospital: Selected Medical Cases. Little, Brown and Co, Boston, 1960, pp vii–ix.

Harvey AM, Bordley J III. Differential Diagnosis: The Interpretation of Clinical Evidence. WB Saunders, Philadelphia, 1955, pp 1–15.

Washburn FA. The Massachusetts General Hospital: Its Development, 1900–1935. Houghton Mifflin, Boston, 1939, pp 115–16.

Zoneraich S. William Dock as I knew him. Am J Cardiol 57:467, 1986.

DIZZY MEDICAL WRITING

To most English-speaking humans on this planet, BM is short for bowel movement. Yet many physicians seem oblivious to this fact and use BM to mean black male. (How would you like to be called a BM?) Depending on one's frame of reference, however, BM also represents bone marrow, basement membrane, basal metabolism, body mass, breast milk, blood monocyte, buccal mass, bachelor of medicine, bacterial meningitis, betamethasone, and biomedical.

–H. L. F. in "DLTBGYD"

DLTBGYD

Ever since my residency training in the mid-1950s, I have enjoyed being a full-time medical educator. Recently, however, I have struggled to maintain a positive attitude. The medicine that I once knew and loved—a proud and noble calling—is crumbling before my very eyes. It has become a big business in which bedside skills and diagnoses are no longer widely appreciated, sought, or even taught. For that reason alone, I was seriously considering retirement. But on my seventieth birthday, a dear friend and colleague gave me a tie emblazoned with the phrase *Non Illegitimi Carborundum.* Those words enabled me to abandon any thought of retirement and serve as my new battle cry.

Speaking of battle cries, I have waged war unsuccessfully for years against abbreviations (AA). Look closely at any medical record or listen carefully to any conversation between health care professionals, and you might understand why—abbreviations abound (AA). In fact, AA "means" Alcoholics Anonymous, African American, adjuvant arthritis, acupuncture anesthesia, allergic alveolitis, alopecia areata, antiarrhythmic agent, or Australia antigen.

The bottom line is this: We tend to forget that the only person who invariably knows what a particular abbreviation stands for is the one who uses it. If AA didn't make the point, perhaps BM will.

To most English-speaking humans on this planet, BM is short for bowel movement. Yet many physicians seem oblivious to this fact and use BM to mean black male. (How would you like to be called a BM?) Depending on one's frame of reference, however, BM also represents bone marrow, basement membrane, basal metabolism, body mass, breast milk, blood monocyte, buccal mass, bachelor of medicine, bacterial meningitis, betamethasone, and biomedical.

When reading patients' charts, I commonly find abbreviations that I have never seen before and cannot for the life of me decipher. One in particular really caught my attention—LGFTD. Who would ever have guessed that LGFTD stands for "Looks good from the door."

Why do physicians abbreviate so much and so often? Partly from habit, but also because it saves time—except for those who try to crack the code. And I think that abbreviating is part of the mystique of our clan, the argot of our lot.

Because of their inescapable ambiguity, abbreviations in medicine can be dangerous, especially when they appear in doctors' orders or prescriptions. If they go unquestioned—and they typically do—the patient can get the wrong test or the wrong medication, and the result can be devastating. Last year in Houston, for example, a nurse misinterpreted an abbreviation in the doctor's orders and gave a patient a fatal dose of potassium intravenously.

Will the pandemic of abbreviations in medicine ever end? Not unless we learn to value clarity and precision over self-serving, thoughtless shortcuts. And not until we concede that abbreviations do nothing for our patients except place them at risk—emotionally, physically, and financially.

By the way. In case you were wondering, *Non Illegitimi Carborundum* is pseudo-Latin for "Don't let the bastards grind you down." Given our penchant for abbreviations, I could save time and space with NIC, but then who would know what I meant? I think I better go with DLTBGYD. If you can't beat 'em, join 'em.

Selected Reading

Daniel TM. The P of the EL is C. J Lab Clin Med 110:127, 1987.
Hurst JW. The art of poor communication. Emory Univ J Med 4:281, 1990.
Stedman's Abbreviations, Acronyms and Symbols, 2nd edn. Lippincott Williams & Wilkins, Baltimore, 1999, p 79.

Dizzy Medical Writing and Editing: No Relief in Sight

This is the sixth presentation of the Dizzy Awards[1-5] honoring baseball's immortal Dizzy Dean. These awards represent excellence in bewildering, unintentionally comical, or downright terrible medical writing—and editing.[6] The recipients, as usual, are excerpts of articles in prominent medical journals.

The Bad Hop Award

"Variceal sclerotherapy is a widely used, effective therapy which causes a variety of pleural, pulmonary and Bacon[10] will be very helpful to clinicians who must evaluate patients with abnormalities related to this procedure."

–Oh where, oh where has my proofreader gone?

The Signs from the Coach Award

"Upon arriving in the emergency room, his vital signs were stable...."

–Did his vital signs arrive by themselves or did he accompany them?

The "Slud into Third" Award

"...if this patient had underwent postmortem examination...."

–That clause should have "underwent" rewording.

The Blooper Award

"As a boy one of my favorite books was Benjamin Franklin's autobiography."

–When the book became a man, did you still like it?

The Squeeze Play Award

"This report describes the case of a young woman with pseudotumor cerebri who herniated after lumbar puncture (LP)."

–How did she get through such a small opening?

The "It Ain't Over Till It's Over" Award

"Despite its rarity, it is known that a real primary mediastinal, sacrococcygeal,[3] or even gonadal[4] teratoma...."

–Say *it* ain't so.

The Batted Out of Order Award

"Sleep oximetry is a simple method for screening patients for nocturnal hypoxaemia which was found to be reliable...."

–Is daytime hypoxaemia equally reliable?

The Make-up Game Award (a tie)

"MR can also evaluate a broad spectrum of muscular dystrophies, neurovascular disorders and metastatic myopathologies."

–My, oh my. Pathologies, pathologies!

"...Whipple's disease may present subclinically or oligosymptomatically...."

–Apparently, it also presents neologicosymptomatically.

The Caught Napping Award

"Because they often present with vague constitutional symptoms, these splenic masses..."

–Don't you just hate it when splenic masses complain?

The Balk Award (a tie)

"To confirm the diagnosis of HPP, SDS-PAGE (sodium dodecyl sulfate-polyacrylamide electrophoresis) is required to demonstrate reduction or lack of alpha I-T80 peptide (domain) of the spectrin molecule [7,8]."

–Quick, turn the GD-PAGE.

"It is suggested that future research in the area of exercise and cognition systematically manipulate the attentional requirements of the tasks selected for the evaluation of cognitive performance."

–Eh?

The "Possibly a Ball, Potentially a Strike" Award

"Given the large number of investigations potentially possible in syncope patients…."

–Maybe perhaps I agree.

The Word Series Award

"These similarities notwithstanding, the toxic oil syndrome was considered a new and distinct clinical entity because none of the conditions or toxicants just mentioned produce the sequential evolution of clinical findings seen among patients with the syndrome: initial respiratory difficulty that resolves over a period of days to weeks only to lead to severe myalgias, persistent eosinophilia, thromboembolic phenomena and late progression to a chronic syndrome involving neuromuscular compromise, sclerodermiform skin changes, joint contractures, chronic hepatopathy and the other manifestations of chronic toxic oil syndrome."

–I got your message, but it took awhile getting here.

The Bag of Soda Pop and Cup of Hot Dog Award (a tie)

"Far from being a trivial symptom, these patients' social and working lives are often limited by abdominal pain and distension...."

–Patients' lives are, indeed, far from being a trivial symptom.

"Although safe in most instances, we present a case report of an individual who had a severe life-threatening complication after this procedure."

–In which instances are your case presentations dangerous?

The Taken Off the Disabled List Award

"There was prompt improvement following the administration of corticosteroids and subsequent recovery."

–What dose of recovery did you administer?

The Screwball Award

"Because of the delayed onset of neurological changes and the cerebrospinal fluid showing reversible symptoms...."

–Since when does spinal fluid show symptoms?

The Batty Title Award (four-way tie)

"Second and Third Responses to the Same Induction Regimen in Relapsing Patients with Multiple Myeloma."

–I have relapsing patience but no relapsing patients.

"Resistant Hypertension in a Tertiary Care Clinic"

–Did you try lowering the clinic's salt intake?

"Major Orthopaedic Surgery on the Leg and Thromboembolism"

–I didn't realize that thromboemboli had bones.

"When Should Patients with Lethal Ventricular Arrhythmia Resume Driving?"

–When they are reincarnated!

The Chit-Chat in the Dugout Award

"However, it should be considered when a patient's history mentions jaundice, hemolytic anemia, and consanguineous parents..."

–When a history speaks, everyone listens.

The Ejected from the Game Award

"The organism was transported to the Centers for Disease Control...."

–Under heavy guard, no doubt.

The Long Fly to the Pitcher Award

"The incidence of renal impairment (one case in each group), hyponatremia (three and four cases, respectively), and other complications (hepatic encephalopathy, gastrointestinal hemorrhage, bacterial infections) after paracentesis, and the clinical course of the disease as estimated by the probability of readmission to hospital during follow-up, causes of readmission, probability of survival, and causes of death were similar in the two groups of patients."

–If you say so.

The Wrong Line-up Award

"A 14-month-old white female infant had a Nissen fundoplication and Janeway gastrostomy done at another institution that failed."

–Was the institution that failed a Savings and Loan?

The Out in Left Field Award

"On secondary survey, the patient's head was atraumatic."

–I recommend a primary survey of that sentence.

The Scorecard Award

"Garrett and Gall (16) in 1953 reported, in an autopsy study, 13 patients with esophageal varices of unknown etiology of 257 cases of varices culled from 18,000 autopsies over a 26-yr period."

–That figures.

The Struckout Twice Award

"Tetanus is a rare disease in the United States, which predominantly affects the elderly and who have a lower prevalence of tetanus immunity compared with younger age groups."

–Words fail me.

The No Hits, No Runs, One Error Award

"Recognition of their manifestations are important, since…."

–It are?

The Illegal Substitution Award

"Thus, an albumin-to-creatinine ratio measured in a single untimed urine specimen is an effective means of identifying diabetic subjects who are at risk of developing overt nephropathy that could replace the more traditional timed urine collections."

–Do you really want to replace urine collections with nephropathy?

The Hall of Shame Award

"…unfortunately, however, not all prostatic nodules are malignant."

–Unfortunately?

References

[1] Fred HL, Robie P. Dizzy medical writing. South Med J 76:1165–66, 1983.

[2] Fred HL, Robie P. Dizzy medical writing: part II. South Med J 77:755–56, 1984.

[3] Fred HL, Robie P. Dizzy medical writing: concluded. South Med J 78:1498–1501, 1985.

[4] Fred HL, Robie P. Dizzy medical writing: report on recent relapses. South Med J 82:897–99, 1989.

[5] Fred HL, Robie P. Dizzy medical writing: will it never end? South Med J 84:755–59, 1991.

[6] Fred HL, Robie P. Dizzy medical editing: causes, consequences, and cures. South Med J 84:760–62, 1991.

Dizzy Medical Writing and Editing: A Decade of Non-Progress*

It's that time again—time to harvest "Dizzies." And this year we have a bumper crop.

A Dizzy is an award honoring the late, great Dizzy Dean, and given for bewildering, unintentionally comical, or downright terrible medical writing and editing.[1-7] The winners are excerpts from recent articles in prominent medical journals.

The Base on Balls Award

"...it should be considered in the differential diagnosis of the acute penis."

–What about the chronic penis?

The Double Play Award

"It appears apparent from the data that the relations between functional cardiac symptoms and panic disorder is worth further examination."

–It certainly do appear apparent.

The Change of Pace Pitch Award

"Three radiologically and bacteriologically confirmed pulmonary tuberculosis patients had eosinophilic pneumonia,...."

–We should leave confirming patients to the clergy.

* Mark Scheid, Ph.D., is coauthor of this article.

The Extra Innings Award

"Since a prospective study of 50 or more HAPE patients would be very hard if not impossible to plan, we had to accept all disadvantages of retrospective data analysis, such as a limited amount of documented information, varying roentgenographic technique and exposure intervals, and last but not least, the selection of patients needing hospital care, ie, probably a more serious subset of subjects with established rather than nascent HAPE studied at low altitude after evacuation."

–It keeps on going and going and going.

The Batted Out of Order Award (a four-way tie)

"In contrast to fractures caused by high-speed trauma, Heyse-Moore and Stoker[5] described a classification of avulsion fractures of the scapula."

–Heyse-Moore and Stoker aren't fractured, but that sentence is.

"While lying on hard surfaces, intramuscular pressures rose to 240 mm Hg,...."

–Intramuscular pressures should always lie on soft surfaces.

"An unusual endobronchial lipoma characterized by pleomorphic, multi-nucleated giant cells admixed with mature adipose cells developed in a 52 year old woman, arising from the right middle lobe bronchus."

–Any woman arising from a bronchus is at risk for being coughed up.

"After 10 years as chairman of medicine, the family moved to California,...."

–The Papa Chair, Mama Chair, and all the little Chairs?

The Trick Play Award

"The disorientation rapidly disappeared while remaining only a discrete dysphasia."

–To disappear yet remain is something that only Houdini could do.

The Fog on the Playing Field Award

"On day 30 he became increasingly vague."

–And on day 31, he disappeared entirely.

The Cases at the Bat Award (a three-way tie)

"...four cases were found to have normal intestinal tracts,...."

"Among ten cases of IA in AIDS in the published literature [6-10], four were granulocytopenic and three...."

"Review of the literature from 1970 to 1990 revealed 37 cases that describe conservative management of spinal epidural abscesses."

–Cases don't have intestinal tracts or granulocytopenia and they can't describe. Patients, however, do.

The Signs from the Coach Award

"Thus, the initial diagnostic FOB in patients with suspected PCP complicating CTD should include BAL and TBLB."

–SOS

The Who's on First, What's on Second Award

"Although there have been several published reports of such infections, all were fatal."

–Thank goodness we didn't read them.

The Full Count Award (a tie)

"Concerning the side-to-side, superoinferior and central-peripheral distribution, there was no change in seven, six, and five patients respectively, whereas five, six and six patients switched between one extreme and balanced distribution and one, one and two patients switched from one extreme to the reverse extreme distribution respectively."

–We're confused for a number of reasons.

"With this category as referent (relative risk = 1.00), relative risks of death associated with losing more than 5 kg, losing between 1 and 5 kg, (more than 1 kg and up to 5 kg) gaining between 1 and 5 kg (more than 1 kg and up to 5 kg), and gaining more than 5 kg were 1.57 (95% confidence interval, 1.34 to 1.84), 1.26 (1.10 to 1.46), 1.06 (0.90 to 1.24), and 1.36 (1.11 to 1.66), respectively."

–Call 911, *stat!*

The Wrong Ballpark Award (a six-way tie)

"A tuberculous abscess secondary to tuberculosis of the spine is a recognized condition (Dawson and Daniell, 1984), though this has never previously been described in the parotid gland."

"There have been a few cases of deep venous thrombosis reported in the lower extremities of athletes [1,6,10]."

"*D. striata,* a parasite of wild cats in the western hemisphere, has been reported in a child."

"Two cases have been described in intravenous drug users and one in a diabetic with a foot wound infection."

"Although mentioned frequently in the literature as a source of absorbable salicylate, Pepto-Bismol use has not been reported in an actual death from salicylate toxicity [9-11]."

"Extrapulmonary pneumocystosis recently has been reported in a number of tissues."

–Cases should be reported in journals, not in glands, athletes' extremities, children, drug users, diabetics, dead people, or tissues.

The Instant Replay Award

"...not all patients are echogenic,..."

–We've got echogenic cousins, nonechogenic uncles, and photogenic wives.

The Odd Player Award

"As a colleague, it is also incumbent to not be too judgmental."

–What kind of a colleague is an "it"?

The Sudden Change in the Line-Up Award (a four-way tie)

"The peritoneum was thickened and hyperemic, with loss of their usual shiny luster."

–"Their" but for the grace of God go "its."

"Another trap is to see the patient when they are heavily medicated...."

–What does "they" have to do with it?

"...if you tell the family that the patient is going to die and they don't, you will never be forgiven."

–What if the family does die?

"We report a 65-yr-old man with hepatitis B virus-related liver cirrhosis and biopsy-proven hepatocellular carcinoma who has undergone spontaneous regression."

–How far back did he go?

The Bad Hop Award (a tie)

"I believe that pulmonary embolism should be suspected and a lung scan should be ordered when patients have a combination of signs, symptoms, and laboratory findings that suggest one of the three &xwhen they occur in patients with evidence of, or predisposition to, venous thromboembolism."

–Someone ought to fix that pothole.

"The pattern found in the chest roentgenogram of the patient whose case was reported was not suggestive of pulmonary involvement by ankylosing spondylitis, and that is the reason because other studies were performed directed to investigate other causes of interstitial pulmonary disease."

–Didn't the roentgenogram show a fractured syntax?

The Caught Out of Position Award

"A 22-year-old woman was admitted in March, 1990, with motor weakness in the limbs and dysphagia."

–It must be awful to have weakness in your dysphagia.

The Babe Ruth Award

"A 14-month-old black female was admitted complaining of abdominal pain and severe constipation during the prior month."

–Out of the mouth of babes...

The Bag of Soda Pop and Cup of Hot Dog Award (a tie)

"However, unlike previous microbiologic studies of *L monocytogenes,* which have been limited to retail foods [8-9], we were able...."

–"We" and "studies" will always be unlike.

"These data are consistent with DeGroote et al., who...."

–Data are consistent with data, not people.

The Bad Call Award

"Although chest pain due to cardiac causes is quite rare,...."

–We couldn't agree less.

The Mixed Signals Award

"Such complications of pneumocococcal infection occurred more or less commonly in the pre-antibiotic era,...."

–Well, which was it? More? or Less?

The Broken Bat Award (a tie)

"Although pulmonary, cutaneous, and genitourinary infections are common in men, splenic abscess and peritoneal infection have rarely been reported in connection with *B. dermatitidis* [1]."

–Could it be because nonsequiturs aren't reportable?

"Tuberculosis had been diagnosed in 1983 (although he had never lived outside the United States),...."

–And he also had never played the tuba, written a novel, or roped a calf.

The Swing and a Miss Award

"The late stroke rate of 3.9 percent over 31 months follow-up with only a 1.8 per cent late stroke rate occurring on the same side as the CEA over 31 months is consistent with published data that documents CEA decreases the risk of stroke within 5 years to 3-6 percent [14,24,25]."

–Three strokes and you're out.

The Bad Road Trip Award

"I am reminded of a memorable case that was discussed [at these infectious disease rounds] of a patient who returned to his home in Los Angeles after vacationing in the desert with sepsis due to *Vibrio*."

–Vacationing in the desert with sepsis is not our idea of fun.

The Scorecard Award (a tie)

"For example, the morning and afternoon results (mean ± SD) were as follows, respectively: for forced vital capacity (FVC), 4.61 ± 0.09 L and 4.71 ± 0.24 L; for FEV_1, 3.75 ± 0.14 L and 3.85 ± 0.13 L; for forced expiratory flow at 25 to 75 percent of FVC (FEF_{25-75}), 3.72 ± 0.40 L/*s* and 3.92 ± 0.37 L/*s*; for total lung capacity (TLC), 6.08 ± 0.23 L and 6.40 ± 0.32 L; and for Dsb, 35.9 ± 3.41 U and 36.1 ± 1.93 U."

"The recurrent *P aeruginosa* group was younger (63 ± 10 vs 74 ± 11 years old [p<0.03]) and spent more time receiving mechanical ventilation (95 ± 64 vs 26 ± 36 days [p<0.01]), in the ICU (101 ± 61 vs 33 ± 35 days [p<0.01]), and in the hospital (144 ± 77 vs 84 ± 32 days [p<0.03])."

–Watch out, the fog's rolling in.

The Hesitation Pitch Award

"The convincing biological and experimental basis, taken together with the initial impressive clinical results on one hand, and the lack of evidence so far for any significant adverse effects on the other hand, single out the addition of dexamethasone to the antibiotic treatment as a new and exciting development in the treatment of acute bacterial meningitis, which should be adopted and further studied at the same time."

–We finally got it, we think.

The Caught Napping Award (a tie)

"Drug testing conducted by the NCAA during the preseason was negative for elicit substances."

–Was the drug testing also negative for *illicit* substances?

"Laboratories should be altered to the possibility of *A hydrophila* as a potential pathogenic organism."

–We prefer to *alert* our laboratories.

The Make-up Game Award

"We evaluated the utility of three recently developed hemostaseologic assays...."

–That sentence lacks logic, hemostaseo or otherwise.

The Win Some, Lose Some Award

"Percutaneous mitral valvotomy resulted in dramatic clinical improvement with complete resolution of liver function."

–The patient lived but his liver died.

The No Hits, No Runs, One Error Award (a four-way tie)

"There are a lack of data regarding how to manage these patients,...."

–Lack of grammar are also a problem.

"Their diagnosis, management, and survival is analyzed."

–They is?

"The frequency and significance of this ECG pattern is not clear."

–They certainly isn't.

"The amount of kilocalorie expenditure needed for health benefit are easy to obtain...."

–Are it?

The Removed from the Line-up Award

"Two months after admission, both legs were amputated below the knee, as well as the thumb."

–Isn't it difficult to amputate legs below the thumb?

The Triple Play Award

"Use of active and active assisted active range of motion is suggested."

–You did it; an active, passive sentence.

The Rookie of the Year Award

"A boy underwent a simple vaginal delivery at term after an uneventful pregnancy."

–Quick! Call the *National Enquirer.*

The Batty Title Award (a seven-way tie)

"Hepatic Resections for Colorectal Metastases in The Netherlands"

–Why resect the liver when the metastases are in The Netherlands?

"Ossification of the Posterior Longitudinal Ligament and Fluorosis"

–There's nothing worse than an ossified fluorosis.

"Peritoneal Tuberculosis: Laparoscopic Patterns and Its Diagnostic Accuracy"

–Is the patterns accurate?

"Natural history of the first non-Q wave myocardial infarction in the placebo arm of the Beta-Blocker Heart Attack Trial"

–Did you hear about the guy whose arm had a heart attack?

"Management and Survival of Meconium Ileus"

–There's nothing sadder than a dead meconium ileus.

"Enterococcal Bacteremia in a Pediatric Institution"

–When institutions with bacteremia have shaking chills, their walls come tumbling down.

"Ectopic Pregnancy in an Urban Teaching Hospital"
–Is that where baby hospitals come from?

The Dean of Dizzies Award

Intergenerational relations are multidimensional in character and their complexity poses problems in conceptualization and measurement, particularly in reference to the current middle-aged population which occupies a unique position relative to their parents' generation.... With the shift from a family system based on consanguine values to one held together by bonds of conjugality and sentiment, the obligations and influences of kinship have been minimized, and the older generation has been placed outside the children's circle of privatized domesticity[3];...."

–Words fail us.

The Battiest Title Award

"On The Proclivity Of The Abductor Fibres Of The Recurrent Laryngeal Nerve To Become Affected Sooner Than The Adductor Fibres, Or Even Exclusively, In Cases Of Undoubted Central Or Peripheral Injury Or Disease Of The Roots Or Trunks Of The Pneumogastric, Spinal Accessory, Or Recurrent Nerves"

–That title appeared more than a century ago, proving that "Dizzies" have been around a long, long time.

References

[1] Fred HL, Robie P. Dizzy medical writing. South Med J 76:1165–66, 1983.

[2] Fred HL, Robie P. Dizzy medical writing: part II. South Med J 77:755–56, 1984.

[3] Fred HL, Robie P. Dizzy medical writing: concluded. South Med J 78:1498–1501, 1985.

[4] Fred HL, Robie P. Dizzy medical writing: report on recent relapses. South Med J 82:897–99, 1989.

[5] Fred HL, Robie P. Dizzy medical writing: will it never end? South Med J 84:755–59, 1991.

[6] Fred HL, Robie P. Dizzy medical editing: causes, consequences, and cures. South Med J 84:760–62, 1991.

[7] Fred HL. Dizzy medical writing and editing: no relief in sight. South Med J 85:743–45, 1992.

Dizzy Medical Editing: Causes, Consequences, and Cures*

> *"Everybody talks about the weather,*
> *but nobody does anything about it."*

So said Mark Twain. Or did he? An alert copy editor would query that quotation and find that it appeared in an unsigned editorial published in the *Hartford Courant* on August 24, 1897.[1] Twenty-four years earlier, that newspaper's editor, Charles Dudley Warner, had collaborated with Mark Twain on *The Gilded Age*.[1] Whether either of these men actually coined the quotation is not our concern here. What does concern us, however, is the ubiquity of copy editing errors we find these days in medical journals, including our own. Though editors and publishers do a lot of talking about this problem, nobody does anything about it—or so it seems.

In another article, we present the fifth in a series of papers on dizzy medical writing. Each of these presentations implies that the authors are solely responsible for the linguistic lapses we cite. We realize, though, that the journals in which the "dizzies" appear are also responsible, particularly the journals' copy editors and proofreaders. Accordingly, we mailed detailed questionnaires to the editorial staffs of 70 prominent American medical journals, seeking their views on why copy editing oversights are so common and how such oversights can be minimized or eliminated. The results of our survey prompt this report.

---

* Pat Robie is coauthor of this article.

Methods and Results

Answers to the questionnaires were anonymous with regard to the respondents' names. Most of the replies, however, arrived in letterhead envelopes. Of the seventy journals contacted, thirty-two responded, including most of the country's largest journals. Table 1 summarizes the responses.

Nearly 60 percent of the respondents added pertinent and pithy comments on how they would like to improve their journals (Table 2). Their suggestions were literate, succinct, and knowledgeable about the need for better editing at all levels. They attributed their problems to many causes, the most common being the lack of time and staff to do the best job possible. That's not surprising because only a small part of the average publishing dollar goes toward manuscript editing. Yet editors—the surrogates of the physician-author—are ultimately responsible for disseminating medical information *accurately*.

TABLE 1. Summary of Copyediting Survey
(70 Questionnaires Mailed; 32 Returned)

1. Job title of respondent:	
Editor, Editor-in-Chief, or Executive Editor	5
Managing Editor, Assistant Managing Editor, Assistant Editor, or Publication Director	8
Director, Editorial Department; Assistant Director, Editorial Processing; Production Coordinator; Freelance Coordinator; Copy Editing Supervisor; Senior Copy Editor; Sr/Manuscript Editor; or Assistant to the Editor	13
Copy Editor	6

2. Number of copy editors the journal normally employs:

Fewer than 5	18	(2 also use freelancers)
5 to 10	9	(1 also uses freelancers)
10 or more	4	(all 4 also use freelancers)
Freelancers only	1	(8/32 use some freelancers)

3. Pages of manuscript the copy editing staff process each year:

Fewer than 2,000	8
2,000 to 5,000	8
5,000 to 10,000	5
10,000 to 20,000	3
More than 50,000	1
No answer	7

4. Comparison of workload per editing staff member with that of 10 years ago:

Heavier	14
Lighter	2
About the same	5
No answer	11

Most said they weren't working there 10 years ago.

5. Statistician reviews statistically based studies (either in-house or as a consultant):

Yes	17
No	5
Sometimes	7
No answer	3

6. A strict distinction exists between those who do "substantive" editing and those who do "copy" editing:

Yes	11	
No	21	Most "no" answers came from small journals.

7. A senior member of the editorial staff reviews the work of junior copy editors:

Routinely	23
When time permits	6
No juniors or no answer	3

8. If anyone (a proofreader, for example) finds an inconsistency or error in a manuscript already approved at a higher level, the correction will be made or the author queried, even if this delays production:

Always	19
Sometimes	12
No answer	1

9. The present copy editing staff is sufficiently large and competent to catch and correct most errors in the manuscripts that pass through the department:

Yes	24
No	8

10. The quality of the writing today compared with that of ten years ago is:

Better	5
Worse	5
Same	10
No response	12

Most said they weren't working there ten years ago.

11. Proportion of manuscripts from major institutions that seem to have had the help of an institutional or author's edition:

Most	4
Some	13
Few	11
No answer	4

12. Current employees of the department meet the level of competency required ten years ago:

Yes	18
No	4
No answer	10

13. Suggestions for improving the quality of copy editing in respondent's department:

Different organization of work	9
More time/more editors	20
More authority for copy editor	5
Other (see Table 2)	12

TABLE 2. Representative Comments from the Respondents

Most of these comments relate to the question of how to improve the quality of copy editing in the respondents' journals. We have paraphrased slightly a few of the comments to preserve the writer's anonymity.

Executive Editor, large specialty journal: Almost all our copy editing is done by regular freelancers. Experienced medical copy editors seem nonexistent, even in Chicago.

Managing Editor, large specialty journal: We don't use a statistician and generally rely on our reviewers to catch mistakes. Some reviewers pay scrupulous attention to statistics; other than that, statistical accuracy is the author's responsibility. Again, some reviewers perform a valuable service in suggesting ways to improve manuscripts. If all reviewers were to give at least some attention to improving poorly written manuscripts, it would help considerably.

Managing Editor, state medical journal: Our staff is so small we all do everything, including proofreading. We have enough editing staff to handle the scientific articles, but the department is expected to handle too many other assignments relating to association business. [Management] doesn't seem to realize that editing a journal is a specialized, full-time job.

Managing Editor, small specialty journal: Our staff is competent—we just need more time to spend on each article. And editing courses and some self-study material on new trends and methods would be helpful.

Senior Copy Editor, medium-sized multidisciplinary journal: Some errors do escape detection—perhaps because we are too rushed (which signifies understaffing). We would benefit from a more complete library of up-to-date reference material.

Copy Editor, large specialty journal: Our copy editors do all types of editing and also do our own proofreading. To do a better job, we need more educational opportunities—courses and workshops on our work, especially for training new copy editors.

Copy Editing Supervisor, large specialty journal: Our management wants faster and faster turnaround times, but this time crunch may result in more errors.

Copy Editing Supervisor, multijournal publishing office: Staff competence is not a problem; the *size* of our staff is not sufficient [to catch all the errors].

Senior Copy Editor, large specialty journal: We need a more extensive review and revision process before manuscripts are accepted for publication; more training in mathematical and technical terminology; more support from chief editors; and more emphasis on quality rather than quantity of editing.

Manuscript Editor, large specialty journal: We need more contact between proofreaders and copy editors so that we can agree on standards. We also need an in-house style and policy manual to use as a reference.

Copy Editor, large multidisciplinary journal: Hiring copy editors with more experience would be a help!

Assistant Director, Editorial Processing, multijournal publishing office: The increased workload and time constraints make most work "rush" and the staff cannot devote the time they need to catch and correct errors. Given these conditions, our error rate remains reasonable, though we have seen an increase in the number of corrections published.

Freelance Coordinator, multijournal office: Turnaround time is too tight to afford time when accuracy should be checked. I don't think we have the competency we did ten years ago because now speed and volume are stressed over quality. Computerization has been both a boon and a bane. Some jobs are easier; others are harder. I think boredom accounts for some of the errors.

Director of Publications, large specialty journal: Our staff needs continuing education opportunities, particularly courses in medical editing.

Copy Editor, medium-sized specialty journal: Our editor accepts manuscripts based on their contribution to medicine, not on whether they are complete or conform to standards. Manuscripts have been accepted that are missing figures and tables, single-spaced, etc. It would be helpful if they were reviewed for conformity to our guidelines before they are accepted. Copy editors do as much substantive editing as time allows and everyone proofreads.

Editor, multijournal publishing office: Use of scanning electronic printers would help prevent errors. Most errors are introduced during printing [typesetting] and are not identified by the authors because of inadequate review of the galley proofs.

Director, Editorial Department, multijournal office: Our copy editors are advised not to do heavy editing unless the journal editor requests it. We take time to correct an error, but not a style inconsistency.

Managing Editor, large specialty journal: We find authors putting results in their Introductions and Comment sections. Errors are often found in the numbers. Numbers in tables don't add up, and we find disagreement between the numbers in the abstract and in the text. Because of these disagreements, I'm led to believe there are also statistical errors in the text (which our staff is not competent to catch). When we make "substantive" changes, we always query the author, and frequently authors don't answer these queries. It would help us tremendously if they would answer all of our questions.

Senior Copy Editor, large multidisciplinary journal: I don't think that [management] appreciates how much time it takes to be *accurate.* The manuscripts we receive have a lot of errors (confusing sentence structure, obvious missing words or even lines, disagreement between different parts of the article concerning figures and even conclusions). Figuring out what the author means takes more time than just marking copy for typesetting, and they really don't want us querying authors anymore because it takes too much time. So a lot of fuzzy writing is getting into print nowadays. I'd like to see fewer articles accepted and more time for getting them right. It is discouraging (and embarrassing) not to have time to do a good job when you know you can do it.

Discussion

The respondents gave a variety of reasons for the proliferation of "howlers" in today's medical literature. In the italicized text that follows, we have distilled their remarks.

Manuscripts don't conform to journal standards / They have missing figures and tables / Errors are found in the numbers / Words or even lines are missing / The results and the conclusions disagree / Authors often fail to answer editorial queries.

Comment. With many notable exceptions, physicians are bad writers. Most spend no time at it, and relatively few ever learn how it should be done. Consequently, even if they *do* read their galley proofs (which many obviously don't), they aren't able to catch their own mistakes, much less those of the editorial staff. For physician-authors wishing to improve their medical writing skills, we recommend generous helpings of Roland,[2] King,[3] Day,[4] and Schwager,[5] topped off with some Bernstein.[6]

We need more time for each article / Management wants faster and faster turnaround times / The time crunch results in more errors / We need more emphasis on quality and less on quantity / It takes time to be accurate.

Comment. Publishers and editors-in-chief formerly demanded literate use of English and realized that excellent editing is an art that isn't compatible with fast turnarounds and high page-per-hour counts. Regrettably, those demands and realizations are less evident today.

Our staff needs more continuing education courses / Some courses on editing and new trends and methods would help / We need a more complete library of reference material / Better training for new copy editors / More training in technical terminology / Hire more experienced copy editors.

Comment. Universities are not turning out the well-rounded scholars they did a generation or two ago, and composition skills are notoriously low, even for arts majors. Moreover, the emphasis throughout a physician's education is on science rather than literature; this face makes the need for good medical editing particularly important. Writing in *Publishers Weekly*, editor-author Jacques Barzun[7] had this to say about copy editing:

> The spread of specialized knowledge, coupled with that of half-education, created a new class of authors— people who knew things of value but wrote badly. For the sake of their information, the publisher in effect appointed a semi-ghost to assist the inarticulate and illiterate. "...first rate stuff but needs a lot of work"—these words are virtually a technical term of the trade.

Our survey indicates that many medical journals are hiring inexperienced copy editors and failing to give them the time and intensive on-the-job training they need—and want. Why don't we hire more experienced copy editors to start with? Because, "Experienced medical copy editors seem nonexistent, even in Chicago," answered the executive editor of a large specialty journal.

Conclusion

Granted, no one can do anything about the weather. But many can do much about bad medical editing (and writing). Those who can do the most are journal sponsors and editors-in-chief. They are the ones ultimately responsible for what comes out in print. And they are the ones who must do more than talk about the problem.

"In medical editing, as in medical practice, being 'almost right' can be dangerous. Absolute accuracy is more than desirable—it is essential."[8]

References

[1] Bartlett's Familiar Quotations, 15th edn, Little, Brown and Co, Boston, 1980, pp 603, 622.

[2] Roland CG. Good Scientific Writing. An Anthology. American Medical Association, Chicago, 1971.

[3] King LS. Why Not Say It Clearly. A Guide to Scientific Writing. Little, Brown and Co, Boston, 1978.

[4] Day RA. How to Write and Publish a Scientific Paper. Oryx Press, Phoenix, Ariz, 1988.

[5] Schwager E. Medical English Usage and Abusage. Oryx Press, Phoenix, Ariz, 1991.

[6] Bernstein TM. The Careful Writer. A Modern Guide to English Usage. Atheneum, New York, 1977.

[7] Barzun J. Behind the blue pencil: censorship or creeping creativity? Publisher's Weekly. September 6, 1985, pp 28–30.

[8] Robie P. Good medical writers and editors are in demand. The Editorial Eye, October 1990, pp 1–2.

MISCELLANY

Those who tell me they prefer the politically correct version could be nonsighted, emotionally different, or committing a categorical inaccuracy. Or, traditionally speaking, they could be blind, crazy, or lying.

–H. L. F. in "On Being Politically Correct"

On Being Politically Correct

In the forty years since I was a junior medical student, much in medicine has changed. Some of the changes I welcome. Others I don't. One of the unwelcomed changes is the recent emphasis on being politically correct in speaking and writing. My feelings on this matter crystallized after I read *The Official Politically Correct Dictionary and Handbook,* by Henry Beard and Christopher Cerf (Villard Books/New York, 1992). The material in that informative and thoroughly referenced work prompted me to compare a theoretical case report written in traditional style with the same report written in politically correct style.

Case Report (Traditional Style)

An eighty-year-old married white woman was brought to the hospital after she became drunk, got lost, and fell into a manhole.

Past history disclosed that her family was poor. Her father had been a janitor during his youth, but later became a vagrant. Her mother worked as a dishwasher. Because both parents were dishonest, they ended up in prison. One brother was mentally retarded and bald. Another brother was a migrant worker. A sister was short, fat, and had never menstruated. An uncle had been accused of killing his wife.

The patient had always been lazy. So, as a girl, she became a prostitute. When that failed, she became homeless.

On physical examination, she smelled of perfume and was intoxicated, nearsighted, and deaf. She also had false teeth and an ugly face.

Shortly after admission, she was found dead in bed.

Case Report (Politically Correct Style)

An eighty-year-chronologically gifted, domestically incarcerated, melanin-impoverished wofem was brought to the hospital after she became sobriety-deprived, got temporarily misoriented, and fell into a personhole.

Past herstory disclosed that her family was economically marginalized. Her father had been an environmental hygienist during his youth, but later became a nonspecifically destinationed individual. Her mother worked as a utensil sanitizer. Because both parents were ethically disoriented, they ended up as clients of the correctional system. One brother was mentally challenged and hair-disadvantaged. Another brother was a seasonal employee. A sister was vertically constrained, horizontally challenged, and had never femstruated. An uncle had been accused of rendering his unpaid sex worker nonviable.

The patient had always been motivationally dispossessed. So, as a prewoman, she became a sex care provider. When that achieved a deficiency, she became involuntarily undomiciled.

On physical examination, she had a discretionary fragrance and was chemically, optically, and aurally inconvenienced. She also had alternative dentation and a cosmetically different face.

Shortly after admission, she was found terminally inconvenienced in bed.

Coda

Those who tell me they prefer the politically correct version could be nonsighted, emotionally different, or committing a categorical inaccuracy. Or, traditionally speaking, they could be blind, crazy, or lying.

Clinical Observations During a 1,000-Mile Footrace

Thinking is more interesting than knowing, but less interesting than looking.
–Goethe

After five stages and 258 miles, I can't move my left foot up or down. Tendinitis has brought me to a standstill. I wait three days, and still I can barely walk, much less run. Greatly disappointed, I withdraw from the Sesquicentennial Trans-Texas Race.[1]

Such was my fate in a race that began at the Texas-New Mexico border on 1 November 1986, and ended twenty-three days later at the San Jacinto Battleground, just past Houston. It spanned 1,044.9 miles, all on major U.S. highways, and consisted of twenty-one pre-deter-mined stages of about fifty miles per day. Two rest days occurred, one each at the end of the first and second weeks.

Of the fourteen starters, two completed the entire course. One of the two *walked* every step of the way, spending twenty to twenty-four hours a day in the process. Four other runners covered more than half of the scheduled mileage. I entered the race solely as a participant, but being the only physician on the scene, I received most of the runners' medical complaints.

The scientific literature on multiday endurance events deals primarily with the biochemical, metabolic, and physiologic consequences;[2-6] it says little about the mental changes[7] and almost nothing about the physical ailments that evolve. Presented here, therefore, are the clinical observations I made during the Trans-Texas run.

Edema: By the second day of the run, swelling of the feet and ankles appeared in about half of the competitors, including me. In some, the swelling progressed and became painful, prompting those afflicted to loosen the laces, slice the heels, and cut out the toes of their shoes. But the swelling persisted and did not abate until the victims stopped running altogether. The eventual winner told me that in a previous 1,000-mile run, he had started in a size 10 shoe but finished in a size 13.

The cause of our swollen feet and ankles is speculative. One probable factor is decreased urinary excretion of sodium with resultant sodium retention and fluid accumulation. Other contributing factors might be tissue damage from the cumulative effect of pounding the concrete and asphalt highways and pooling of fluid in the extremities from being upright ten to twenty or more hours a day. The swelling itself might have impaired venous and lymphatic drainage from the feet, thus perpetuating or even increasing the swelling.

Edema of the lower legs and ankles has appeared in other runners after completing an ultramarathon.[8] It has also appeared, along with facial edema, in five semi-sedentary men who completed seven consecutive days of strenuous hill-walking.[6] Studies of water balance and distribution in those five men showed that during exercise, the packed cell volume fell, reaching a maximum of 11 percent by day five; sodium retention reached a cumulative maximum of 358 mmol by day six; and no change occurred in the arginine vasopressin levels or in the serum electrolyte concentrations. The plasma volume and interstitial fluid volume increased, however, and the intracellular fluid volume decreased in all participants.

Facial swelling, especially of the eyelids, also occurred in every runner early in our race. In some it was striking. At first, I attributed this swelling to running directly into freezing rain and strong winds during the first four days of the race. But our hands and forearms also swelled, a finding that I attributed initially to having our arms hang down most of the day. Yet all of the swelling continued after the weather improved and did not diminish after we rested at night. I believe, therefore, that the swelling of our eyelids, forearms, and hands—like the swelling of our feet and ankles—resulted primarily from sodium retention. Wherever it appeared, the edema remained until three or four days after the athletes stopped running completely. The lag time for the swelling to disappear might reflect how long it takes for complex hormonal responses[9] and altered renal function to return to normal and for tissue damage to resolve after exertion ends.

Tendons: Tendinitis ultimately developed in half of the contestants. The affected tendons were thickened, tender, and warm, and painful on movement of the foot. Crepitus along the tendon sheath was also evident in four of the athletes. Intense inflammation of the extensor hallucis longus, extensor digitorum longus, and anterior tibial tendons sidelined me and two other runners. Achilles tendinitis appeared in four runners, persisting throughout the race in two, including the winner. It disappeared in the other two despite their continued running.

The mechanism by which tendinitis occurred is unclear. I believe that as our feet got bigger, our tight shoes squeezed the tendons of our feet and ankles. The squeezing, in turn, impeded free movement of the tendons within their sheaths, leading to further irritation and swelling. Continued running for unusually long distances, especially over hard surfaces whose slant and grade were frequently changing, clearly worsened and may have been the prime cause of the problem.

Muscles: Surprisingly, muscle ailments were mild and inconsequential. Although every participant was tired and stiff at the end of each run, zip and flexibility returned routinely the next morning. Indeed, with three consecutive weeks of fifty miles a day to run, we couldn't afford to go "all out." We were pacing, not racing. This approach may have minimized muscle breakdown.

Joints: Two runners manifested swollen knees seventy-two hours into the race. In one, the swelling was bilateral, minimal, and fleeting; the knees were slightly tender. In the other runner, one knee swelled to twice the size of its mate; the enlargement was symmetric, without redness or heat. Because the affected knee was pain free, however, the athlete—a national record-holder in the forty-eight-hour run—opted to continue. For the next 400 miles, the swelling did not change. Then, inexplicably, it began to subside. As the runner covered an additional 200 miles, the swelling disappeared entirely, and never returned. Incredible!

The genesis of the swollen knees is conjectural. Bilateral Achilles tendinitis preceded the onset of knee complaints in both runners. Perhaps, then, the pain from the tendinitis led to an altered running style, thereby increasing the stress to the knees.

Mental: All contestants agreed that running day after day on major highways, often under brutal weather conditions, was as stressful mentally as it was physically. Furthermore, the inept planning and woefully deficient support services from those in charge of the race placed additional hardships, both mental and physical, on the runners.

Trying to run fifty miles every day left us little time to eat, bathe, or sleep. To complicate matters, getting enough food during and after each run was a constant problem. We never had time to wash or dry our clothes. And no one ever seemed to know until the last minute whether we had a place to sleep each night, and if we did, where and what kind it would be.

Each stage was too far for most of the runners to cover in daylight. Consequently, we often ran at night—sometimes all night. Far worse, we had no protection against traffic and soon learned that we couldn't afford to stumble, weave, or lose our concentration.

One misstep could be our last. Wind gusts from passing eighteen-wheelers blew us off our feet and deposited us as much as five yards down the way. And our eyes played tricks on us. You think, for example, you see a support van, but it turns out to be a bush. You think you see a sign in the distance, but it turns out to be an oncoming truck. Getting lost was a continuous possibility, and most of the runners did so at one time or another. These difficulties and the threat of being injured or killed multiplied exponentially at night.

A previous report has described an organic mental disorder associated with prolonged competitive stress.[7] Memory deficits, difficulty in tasks of recall and retention, and episodic visual hallucinations appeared in persons who completed an Alaskan dog sled race that spanned 1,049 miles and entailed two to four weeks of intense physical exertion, periods of sleep deprivation, and exposure to extreme cold.

Miscellaneous: Three runners suffered hypothermia; two had food poisoning; and one experienced severely infected toes. None of these complications stopped the affected individuals. On day four, the eventual winner developed a large area of stiffness, pain, and swelling along with heat and redness over the left side of his back. It persisted throughout the race. I suspect the ailment resulted from the way he positioned his shoulders and swung his arms as he ran. Sadly, but not unexpectedly, one runner fell prey to a hit-and-run driver at night. The accident left him with a crushed humerus and functionless arm.

These observations permit me three conclusions and two hopes:

The conclusions: participants in multiday races would do well to bring along extra shoes larger than those they ordinarily wear; tendinitis is the injury most likely to stop a runner in such races; and no matter how well organized or supported, footraces on U.S. thoroughfares carry an inordinate risk to life and limb.

The hopes: that someday we will fully understand what causes swelling of the eyelids, forearms, hands, feet, and ankles during multiday endurance events; and what causes a knee to swell massively, undergo 400 miles of hard running, then gradually return to its normal size during 200 additional miles of running.

References

[1] Fred HL. Observations (medical and otherwise) from the Trans-Texas Race. Ultrarunning 6(8):12–14, 1987.

[2] Dressendorfer RH, Wade CE, Keen CL, Scaff JH Jr. Plasma mineral levels in marathon runners during a 20-day road race. Phys Sportsmed 10:113–18, 1982.

[3] Peters AJ, Dressendorfer RH, Rimer J, Keen CL. Diets of endurance runners competing in a 20-day road race. Phys Sportsmed 14:63–70, 1986.

[4] Lathan SR, Cantwell JD. A run for the record: Studies on a trans-American ultramarathon. JAMA 245:367–68, 1981.

[5] Jobin J, Tremblay A, Samson P. Effect of a 6,400-km run on a 60-year-old man. Phys Sportsmed 12:53–61, 1984.

[6] Williams ES, Ward MP, Milledge JS, et al. Effect of the exercise of seven consecutive days hill-walking on fluid homeostasis. Clin Sci 56:305–16, 1979.

[7] Popkin MK, Stillner V, Pierce CM. Organic mental disorder associated with prolonged competitive stress. Compr Psychiatry 22:522–27, 1981.

[8] Fred HL. The 100-mile run: preparation, performance, and recovery. A case report. Am J Sports Med 9:258–61, 1981.

[9] Francesconi RP. Endocrinological responses to exercise in stressful environments. *In* Exercise and Sports Sciences Reviews, American College of Sports Medicine Series, Vol 16. Macmillan Publishing Company, New York, 1988, pp 255–84.

On An Average Day

What does the average American buy, eat, watch, read, cook, and spend on an average day? And how does that compare with similar activities in the former Soviet Union? You can find out for $13.90—the aggregate cost of two books by Tom Heymann. One of them, published in 1989, deals with America; its title is *On An Average Day*. The other, published in 1990, is titled *On An Average Day in the Soviet Union*. (Both books are available through Fawcett Columbine, New York.)

These paperback volumes offer detailed information on a wide range of topics, including health care. Did you know, for example, that on an average day in our country, 10,500 babies are born—2,000 to unwed mothers and 178 from artificial insemination? Among these births are 217 sets of twins and 5 sets of triplets. At the other end, 8,000 Americans join the American Association of Retired Persons (AARP); 3,500 enter nursing homes; and 6,000 die: 1,200 from cancer and almost twice that number from heart disease.

On an average day, Americans pay a whopping $1 1/4 billion for health care—approximately $550 million to hospitals, $290 million to doctors, $120 million to nursing homes, $93 million to dentists, $45 million for prescription drugs, $11 million for over-the-counter pain relievers, and $1 1/3 million for laxatives. Also on an average day, 37 million Americans don't have health insurance coverage; 2,700 lose it; and another 2,700 are denied routine health care because they cannot pay.

If the preceding figures don't whet your appetite or otherwise arouse you, try these: on an average day, Americans consume 24 1/2 million hot dogs; eat 2 3/4 million Dunkin' Donuts; drink 524 million servings of Coca-Cola; spend $10 1/2 million on potato chips; and buy one million condoms, almost half purchased by women.

In the Soviet Union on an average day, 15,300 babies are born—1,500 to unmarried women. Among these births are 122 sets of twins and one set of triplets. Additionally, 7,700 Soviets die, 4,200 from heart disease and 1,250 from cancer. There are 18,000 rural Soviet hospitals, of which 11,700 have no hot water, 4,800 have no sewage systems, and 3,000 have no running water.

Consider, too, that on an average day, 70 million Soviets smoke; 21 million are alcoholics; 15 million suffer from psychiatric illness; six million are homosexuals; two million are drug abusers; and 10,000 carry the AIDS virus. The government spends $96 1/2 million on health care and produces 600,000 condoms, 2 1/2 million short of the daily demand.

On an average day in America *and* in the Soviet Union, no one would read this editorial.

Parliament of Whores

> I have only one firm belief about the American political system, and that is this: God is a Republican and Santa Claus is a Democrat.
>
> God is an elderly or, at any rate, middle-aged male, a stern fellow, patriarchal rather than paternal, and a great believer in rules and regulations. He holds men strictly accountable for their actions. He has little apparent concern for the material well-being of the disadvantaged. He is politically connected, socially powerful, and holds the mortgage on literally everything in the world. God is difficult. God is unsentimental. It is very hard to get into God's heavenly country club.
>
> Santa Claus is another matter. He's cute. He's nonthreatening. He's always cheerful. And he loves animals. He may know who's been naughty and who's been nice, but he never does anything about it. He gives everyone everything they want without thought of a quid pro quo. He works hard for charities, and he's famously generous to the poor. Santa Claus is preferable to God in every way but one: There is no such thing as Santa Claus.

Those words close the preface of an intriguing book that "attempts to explain the entire U.S. government." The book is titled *Parliament of Whores,* by P. J. O'Rourke (Atlantic Monthly Press, New York, 1991). On the dust cover, former President Richard Nixon says, "Whether you agree with P. J. O'Rourke or not...he writes a helluva piece." That he does. Offering enlightenment through humor, the author rivets his readers throughout, ending as he began—with a bang:

> Authority has always attracted the lowest elements in the human race. All through history mankind has been bullied by scum. Those who lord it over their fellows and toss commands in every direction and would boss the grass in the meadow about which way to bend in the wind are the most depraved kind of prostitutes. They will submit to any indignity, perform any vile act, do anything to achieve power. The worst off-sloughings of the planet are the ingredients of sovereignty. Every government is a parliament of whores.
>
> The trouble is, in a democracy the whores are us.

The timeliness and relevance of *Parliament of Whores* are striking, considering that the book appeared shortly before the Senate confirmation hearings on Judge Clarence Thomas. That real-life spectacle provided an in-depth, on-the-scene look at our government in action. It enabled each of us to judge the way members of the Senate Judiciary Committee examine and cross-examine witnesses. It spurred most of us to draw conclusions about each senator's competence, compassion, and candor. And it stimulated me to wonder what would happen if physicians, rather than U.S. senators, had to do their work under the scrutiny of television cameras.

Fantasize with me for a moment. A committee of high-ranking physicians has the responsibility of confirming the physical and mental fitness of, for example, a Presidential nominee. The job calls for each physician to elicit the nominee's medical history and to do whatever physical examination seems appropriate. These activities, normally done in the privacy of the doctor's office, unfold instead before a worldwide television audience. Imagine the public's response!

Don't worry. It's only fantasy—at least for now.

Cause or Coincidence?

For me, the MD after my name means more than "medical doctor." It means "making decisions."[1] And making correct medical decisions requires an ability to distinguish between cause and coincidence. That ability, in turn, requires knowledge of the pathogenesis and natural history of diseases. Without such knowledge, the practitioner "...flounders along in an aimless fashion, never able to gain any accurate conception of disease, practising a sort of popgun pharmacy, hitting now the malady and again the patient, he himself not knowing which."[2] Consider the following three coincidences, two of which masqueraded as causes.

CASE 1. In the early 1960s, I helped care for a young boy who had sickle cell disease and a serum bilirubin concentration of 100 mg/dL. During the first three weeks of hospitalization, his intense hy-perbilirubinemia fluctuated only minimally. As a last-ditch measure to avoid exploratory celiotomy, we ordered a trial of empiric steroid therapy. Within twenty-four hours, his serum bilirubin concentration began to fall, and by the end of a week, it had dropped to near-normal levels. We immediately assumed that the steroid therapy caused his miraculous improvement. But then we discovered that because of a clerical error, the patient never received the steroids. Though we did not determine why the serum bilirubin concentration fell so abruptly, this case taught me how easy it is to draw wrong conclusions and how common it is for doctors to take credit for something Mother Nature has done.

CASE 2. In 1991, the house officers asked me to see a young man with epilepsy whom they believed had developed aspiration pneumonia after a seizure. They had given him antibiotics because his admission chest film demonstrated infiltrates confined to the upper lobes. Twelve hours into his hospital course, a repeat chest film showed partial clearing of the infiltrates; by the next day, the chest film was normal. The house officers concluded that the antibiotics had caused the roentgenographic improvement and that such improvement implied infection.[3] They were not aware that aspiration pneumonia virtually never appears solely in *both* upper lobes. They also did not know that aspiration pneumonia does not resolve completely within twenty-four hours—with or without antibiotic therapy. And they were not familiar with postictal pulmonary edema,[4] the correct diagnosis in this case. Had they not shown the patient to me or to another senior clinician, they never would have recognized their error.

CASE 3. In 1984, my wife and I were 10,000 miles from Houston, in Xian, China, a city of three million people. As we stepped into the crowded elevator of our hotel, someone said, "Hi, Herb." Looking up, I saw a friend of ours standing in the elevator. He, too, was from Houston. Meeting him there was a coincidence—I think.

References

[1] Fred HL. MD. South Med J 71:887, 1978.

[2] Osler W. Teaching and thinking. *In* Aequanimitas: With Other Addresses to Medical Students, Nurses and Practitioners of Medicine, 2nd edn. P Blakiston's Son & Co, Philadelphia, 1906, p 127.

[3] Kim JH, Gallis HA. Observations on spiraling empiricism: its causes, allure, and perils, with particular reference to antibiotic therapy. Am J Med 87:201–206, 1989.

[4] Huff RW, Fred HL. Postictal pulmonary edema. Arch Intern Med 117:824–28, 1966.

There but for the Grace of God...

We Americans have much to complain about. Our economy is struggling, our health care structure is sagging, our crime rate is soaring—now Rubbergate and the Rodney King matter. Before we complain, however, we ought to look around. A case in point is that of my friend, Jim, a Houston attorney who wrote me the following letter.

January 30, 1992

Dear Herb,

This letter is purely personal; however, you might wish to show it to a friend the next time he complains about the economy.

At approximately 7 A.M. last October 7, I walked out to my back alley, where I was confronted by a large man with a gun. He requested that I take him into my house, but I refused, because I was afraid he might kill my wife and our maid. So I turned and ran away from the house, hoping that he would chase me. Instead, he shot me. The bullet lodged in my spine and knocked me facedown onto the concrete. I don't remember much after that, except that my head swelled to the size of a pumpkin. I was taken to the local trauma hospital, where I was "stabilized."

Late that evening, I was transferred to a private hospital. After I had spent several days in the intensive care unit, the bullet was removed, and I was "stabilized" again. You might think that was enough, but the force of the blow to my face when I hit the concrete made it necessary for me to have fragments of bone transplanted from my hip to the back of my eye socket. Now, you'd think that would surely be enough, wouldn't you? But, no. While I was in the intensive care unit being "stabilized," my heart, for whatever reason, decided to "arrest." It stopped working for over an hour. Fortunately, two of the best cardiologists in the medical center were standing nearby, and after 15 shock treatments, my heart started beating again. I was "stabilized" once more, and after spending two weeks in the coronary care unit, I was sent to a place down the street for rehabilitation.

On the night of December 31, my wife and I and another couple were celebrating New Year's Eve by playing a dignified game of dominos in my hospital room. Suddenly, my eyes rolled back, and I began to have some sort of seizure. My wife and good friends thought that I was celebrating too exuberantly, but that wasn't the case. In reality—if by now you can still grant me any veracity—my heart had stopped again.

Help was called for, and someone came running down the hall and began beating on me. Soon thereafter, an ambulance took me four blocks down the way to an acute care hospital, where I remain, confined to a wheelchair at best. Incidentally, that ambulance ride cost me $300, even though it is my understanding that someone was beating on me the whole bumpy ride.

Due to the excellent efforts of my cardiologists and nurses, I have been brought back to life and "stabilized" several times. Now, I am kept alive by the use of chemicals. My doctors tell me that something must be done to stop my heart from stopping. Unfortunately, extensive testing and another "arrest" have left me with only two options—a heart transplant or continued attempts to control the tachycardia and arrhythmia problems through the use of chemicals. Neither alternative is appealing, but I find the transplant option the more favorable.

No matter what the next chapter may hold, I want to say to all my many friends how much their prayers, flowers, cards, and calls have meant to me. I am truly blessed by such friendship. And I am doubly blessed to have a mother, a wife, and six children who love me deeply and who have supported me throughout this ordeal.

For having read this rather lengthy epistle, you surely need to give your own heart "a rest."

Sincerely,

Jim

Shortly after this article appeared in print, Jim received the heart of a fifteen-year-old girl. Now, ten years post transplant, he remains active and forever grateful.

C. T. Scanner Dies

Advances in medical technology have greatly enhanced our capacity to render optimum patient care. But at the same time, these advances have shifted the emphasis of medical practice from the bedside to the laboratory. Consequently, managing numbers, rather than the patients who own the numbers, is fast becoming the norm.

Each of us sees cases in which the numbers live but the patient dies. In such instances, we typically attribute the death to forces beyond our control and give no further thought to the matter. Yet what about the cases in which the patient lives but the *numbers* die?

The other day, for example, the house officers showed me a patient who was being kept in the intensive care unit solely because the results of her blood gas analyses were repeatedly abnormal. The patient, however, looked fairly well, and her condition was stable. So I recommended that we let the blood gas numbers pass away and let the patient recover at home. We did, and she did.

That incident made me wonder how the obituary might read if a test or gadget died. I then fantasized the following:

> C. T. Scanner, prominent member of the laboratory group at Have Scanner Will Image Hospital, met his maker (General Electric) yesterday after a long but lucrative battle against overuse and overreliance. When the end came, "Cat Scan," as he was fondly known throughout the world, was surrounded by his sister Spiral, his brother Electron-Beam, and his two cousins M. R. Imaging and M. R. Angiography.

Death of this marvelous tool has left the medical community in a shambles. Activity at the hospital has slowed to a standstill, and revenue has plummeted. Even worse, physicians must now talk with and examine the patients.

Pallbearers will be Cat Scan's overordered and overrelied on colleagues, including E. Rythrocyte Sedrate, C. Rum Tumormarkers, O. Twosat Uration, and B. Lood Gas. Burial will take place at the landfill south of the city with I. M. Heartbroken, Chief Radiologist, officiating. Donations in memory of Cat Scan should be sent to the hospital's emergency relief fund or to a health maintenance organization of your choice.

No one can dispute the value of today's medical technology. And no one can deny that such technology has triggered a spate of indiscriminate and exorbitantly expensive testing and treatment. To counter this negative effect of high-tech medicine, we need to restore some of the high-touch medicine of yesteryear. If we do, we and our patients will be a lot better off.

EPILOGUE

Epilogue

In 1929, the year of my birth, house calls were part of a doctor's daily routine. I can still remember times as a youngster when the family doctor came to my sickbed to examine and comfort me. If his schedule permitted, he would stay to have a meal with my parents or play cards with my dad. On Sundays, he often came by just to visit. We adored him, and he adored us.

Unfortunately, the practice of making house calls gradually waned, and by the time I entered medical school in 1950, it had largely disappeared. Nevertheless, ties between patients and their doctors remained strong until the 1970s, when advanced in medical technology began burgeoning. As a result, high-tech medicine began replacing the high-touch medicine that I grew up with and loved.

For three decades now, I have watched with sadness the progressive demise of bedside medicine. That sadness, in turn, has provoked many of the essays assembled here.

What can we expect of medicine in this new millennium? I briefly addressed that question some years ago:

> Overreliance on modern technology is undermining the physician's use of his mind and five senses for diagnoses. Jumping from the patient's chief complaint to a host of tests and procedures is commonplace. And when that approach does not work, the physician simply orders more tests or seeks consultation. This malady of practice is making the skilled clinical diagnostician a vanishing species. It is taking much of the fun and challenge out of medicine. It is

> depersonalizing the doctor-patient relationship. Even worse, it threatens the individuality of patient care.
>
> The day could come when physicians per se will no longer be necessary. In their place will be the ultimate gimmick—a convenience-store computer that takes care of your medical needs and tells your fortune, all for a quarter.[1]

Later on, I added: "By moving from the bedside to the laboratory, we are becoming proficient in ordering tests, but deficient in taking a pertinent medical history and doing a good physical examination. As a clinician and as a patient, I find that tradeoff uneven and unfortunate."[2]

Looking back on my professional career, I see enormous progress in our ability to detect and treat disease. But along with that progress, we have sacrificed to a large extent the very core of doctoring—humanism. We need to recapture the Oslerian spirit and strive diligently to promote and preserve the human element in medicine. Reaching that goal will require doctors with commitment, compassion, candor, and common sense. Doctors who can look at, listen to, and talk with their patients. Doctors who understand that medicine is a calling, not a business. And doctors who always put the patient first. In short—doctors who practice medicine the old-fashioned way.

References

[1] Fred, HL. Elephant Medicine—and More: Musings of a Medical Educator. Mercer University Press, Macon, Georgia, 1988, pp 82–83.

[2] Fred, HL. Say Aah (Hah): A Medical Educator Mouths Off. Mercer University Press, Macon, Georgia, 1991, pp 53–65.